THE CORE COMPETEN(
IN HOSPITAL MEDICI
A Framework for Curriculum Develop
By the Society of Hospital Medicine

T0280759

Editors

Michael J. Pistoria, DO, FACP
Associate Program Director, Internal Medicine Program
Medical Director, Hospitalist Services
Lehigh Valley Hospital
Allentown, PA
Assistant Professor of Medicine
The Pennsylvania State University College of Medicine
Hershey, PA

Alpesh N. Amin, MD, MBA, FACP
Executive Director, Hospitalist Program
Vice Chair for Clinical Affairs and Quality, Department of Medicine
Associate Program Director, Internal Medicine Residency
Medicine Clerkship Director
University of California, Irvine
Orange, CA

Daniel D. Dressler, MD, MSc
Director, Hospital Medicine Services
Emory University Hospital
Assistant Professor of Medicine
Emory University School of Medicine
Atlanta, GA

Sylvia C. W. McKean, MD
Medical Director
Brigham and Women's Faulkner Hospitalist Service
Assistant Professor of Medicine
Harvard Medical School
Boston, MA

Tina L. Budnitz, MPH
Senior Advisor for New Initiatives
Society of Hospital Medicine
Philadelphia, PA

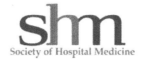

Society of Hospital Medicine

This work was originally published as a supplement to the *Journal of Hospital Medicine* (Volume 1, Supplement 1, 2006)

ISBN: 9780470931479

The *Journal of Hospital Medicine* (Print ISSN 1553-5592; online ISSN 1553-5606 at Wiley InterScience, www.interscience.wiley.com) is published bimonthly, one volume per year, for the Society of Hospital Medicine by Wiley Subscription Services, Inc., a Wiley Company, 111 River Street, Hoboken, NJ 07030. Periodicals postage pending at Hoboken, NJ, and at additional mailing offices. Subscription price (Volume 1, 2006): Complimentary online access to *Journal of Hospital Medicine* will be available to all institutions who register for access. Personal rate: $110.00. All subscriptions containing a print element shipped outside US will be sent by air. Payment must be made in US dollars drawn on a US bank. Claims for undelivered copies will be accepted only after the following issue has been delivered. Please enclose a copy of the mailing label. Missing copies will be supplied when losses have been sustained in transit and where reserve stock permits. Please allow four weeks for processing a change of address. For subscription inquiries, please call (201) 748-6645 or e-mail: SUBINFO@wiley.com.

Postmaster: Send address changes to *Journal of Hospital Medicine,* Subscription Distribution, John Wiley & Sons, Inc., 111 River Street, Hoboken, NJ 07030.

Advertising Sales: Inquiries concerning advertising should be directed to: (display advertising) Patrice Culligan, National Account Manager, (212) 904-0369, pculligan@pminy.com; (recruitment) Robert Zwick, Classified Advertising Manager, (212) 904-0377, rzwick@pminy.com; Pharmaceutical Media Inc., 30 East 33rd Street, 4th Floor, New York, NY 10016.

Reprints: Reprint sales and inquiries should be directed to the Customer Service Department, John Wiley & Sons, Inc., 111 River Street, Hoboken, NJ 07030. Tel: (201) 748-8789.

Other correspondence: Address all other correspondence to: *Journal of Hospital Medicine,* Publisher, John Wiley & Sons, Inc., 111 River Street, Hoboken, NJ 07030.

Instructions for Authors for preparation of manuscript appear online at http://www.interscience.wiley.com/jhm.

∞ **This paper meets the requirements of ANSI/NISO Z39.48-1992 (Permanence of Paper).**

THE CORE COMPETENCIES IN HOSPITAL MEDICINE
A Framework for Curriculum Development by the Society of Hospital Medicine

TABLE OF CONTENTS

Acknowledgement v
Editors and Contributors vii
Introduction xv

Section 1: CLINICAL CONDITIONS

1.1	Acute Coronary Syndrome	2
1.2	Acute Renal Failure	4
1.3	Alcohol and Drug Withdrawal	6
1.4	Asthma	8
1.5	Cardiac Arrhythmia	10
1.6	Cellulitis	12
1.7	Chronic Obstructive Pulmonary Disease	14
1.8	Community-Acquired Pneumonia	16
1.9	Congestive Heart Failure	18
1.10	Delirium and Dementia	20
1.11	Diabetes Mellitus	22
1.12	Gastrointestinal Bleed	24
1.13	Hospital-Acquired Pneumonia	26
1.14	Pain Management	28
1.15	Perioperative Medicine	30
1.16	Sepsis Syndrome	32
1.17	Stroke	34
1.18	Urinary Tract Infection	36
1.19	Venous Thromboembolism	38

Section 2: PROCEDURES

2.1	Arthrocentesis	42
2.2	Chest Radiograph Interpretation	44
2.3	Electrocardiogram Interpretation	45
2.4	Emergency Procedures	47
2.5	Lumbar Puncture	50
2.6	Paracentesis	52
2.7	Thoracentesis	54
2.8	Vascular Access	56

Section 3:   HEALTHCARE SYSTEMS

3.1   Care of the Elderly Patient... 60
3.2   Care of Vulnerable Populations.. 62
3.3   Communication 63
3.4   Diagnostic Decision Making 65
3.5   Drug Safety, Pharmacoeconomics and Pharmacoepidemiology...... 66
3.6   Equitable Allocation of Resources.. 68
3.7   Evidence Based Medicine 69
3.8   Hospitalist as Consultant... 71
3.9   Hospitalist as Teacher.. 72
3.10   Information Management 75
3.11   Leadership.. 76
3.12   Management Practices 79
3.13   Nutrition and the Hospitalized Patient 81
3.14   Palliative Care... 82
3.15   Patient Education 85
3.16   Patient Handoff 87
3.17   Patient Safety 88
3.18   Practice Based Learning and Improvement..................................... 91
3.19   Prevention of Healthcare-Associated Infections and Antimicrobial Resistance.... 92
3.20   Professionalism and Medical Ethics 94
3.21   Quality Improvement... 97
3.22   Risk Management... 98
3.23   Team Approach and Multidisciplinary Care.................................... 99
3.24   Transitions of Care.. 100

APPENDICES

I. Abbreviations   101

II. Organizations Cited in Text   102

III. Core Competencies in Hospital Medicine: Development and Methodology   103
*Daniel D. Dressler, Michael J. Pistoria, Tina L. Budnitz, Sylvia C. W. McKean, and
Alpesh N. Amin*
Reprinted from *Journal of Hospital Medicine,* Volume 1, Number 1, 2006, Pages 48–56

IV. How to Use the Core Competencies in Hospital Medicine: A Framework for   113
Curriculum Development
*Sylvia C. W. McKean, Tina L. Budnitz, Daniel D. Dressler, Alpesh N. Amin, and
Michael J. Pistoria*
Reprinted from *Journal of Hospital Medicine,* Volume 1, Number 1, 2006, Pages 57–67

ACKNOWLEDGEMENT

The development of *The Core Competencies* would not have been possible without the support and assistance of the Society of Hospital Medicine staff and countless practicing Hospitalists across the United States. The editors thank Parmanand Singh for research assistance, Lillian Higgins for project coordination, and Dr. Daniel Budnitz for assistance with medical editing and chapter formatting. Kathryn Alexander deserves special thanks for her medical editing and expertise and mix of patience and persistence that brought this project to completion. The editors also thank their families for all their patience and support throughout the development process.

Society of Hospital Medicine leadership and subject matter experts who provided content, review and guidance include:

Preetha Basaviah, MD
Jasminka Criley, MD
Douglas Cutler, MD
Steve Embry, MD
Christine Faulk, MD
Scott Flanders, MD

Jeffrey Genato, MD
Jeanne Huddleston, MD
Jennifer Kleinbart, MD
David Likosky, MD
Frank Michota, MD
Kevin O'Leary, MD

Michael Rovzar, MD
Winthrop Whitcomb, MD
Kevin Whitford, MD
Dorothea Wild, MD
Mitch Wilson, MD

SHM Benchmarks Committee
SHM Education Committee
SHM Geriatrics Task Force
SHM Health Quality Patient
   Safety Committee

SHM Non Physician Providers
   Task Force
SHM Pediatrics Committee
SHM Ethics Committee
SHM Executive Board of
   Directors

SHM Leadership Committee
SHM Palliative Care Task Force
SHM Pediatrics Core Curriculum
   Task Force

EDITORS

Michael J. Pistoria, DO, FACP
    Associate Program Director, Internal Medicine Program; Medical Director, Hospitalist Services
    Lehigh Valley Hospital, Allentown, PA
    Assistant Professor of Medicine, The Pennsylvania State University College of Medicine
    Hershey, PA

Alpesh N. Amin, MD, MBA, FACP
    Executive Director, Hospitalist Program
    Vice Chair for Clinical Affairs and Quality, Department of Medicine
    Associate Program Director, Internal Medicine Residency
    Medicine Clerkship Director
    University of California, Irvine
    Orange, CA

Daniel D. Dressler, MD, MSc
    Director, Hospital Medicine Services, Emory University Hospital
    Assistant Professor of Medicine, Emory University School of Medicine
    Atlanta, GA

Sylvia C.W. McKean, MD
    Medical Director, Brigham and Women's Faulkner Hospitalist Service
    Assistant Professor of Medicine, Harvard Medical School
    Boston, MA

Tina L. Budnitz, MPH
    Senior Advisor for New Initiatives
    Society of Hospital Medicine
    Philadelphia, PA

CONTRIBUTORS

Richard Albert, MD
    Professor of Medicine, University of Colorado Health Science Center
    Adjunct Professor of Engineering and Computer Science, University of Denver
    Chief of Medicine, Denver Health Medical Center
    Denver, CO
    Equitable Allocation of Resources

Leland Allen, MD
    Chief of Infectious Diseases
    Shelby Baptist Medical Center
    Birmingham, AL
    Hospital-Acquired Pneumonia

Alpesh Amin, MD, MBA, FACP
    Executive Director, Hospitalist Program
    Vice Chair for Clinical Affairs and Quality, Department of Medicine
    Associate Program Director, Internal Medicine Residency
    Medicine Clerkship Director
    University of California, Irvine
    Orange, CA
    Asthma

Jeffrey Barsuk, MD
    Assistant Professor of Medicine
    Northwestern University
    Chicago, IL
    Thoracentesis

Stephen Bartold, MD, FACP
> Associate Professor of Medicine
> Texas Tech University
> Odessa, TX
> *Information Management*

Lee Biblo, MD
> Professor and Vice Chairman, Department of Medicine
> Medical College of Wisconsin
> Milwaukee, WI
> *Electrocardiogram Interpretation*

Daniel Budnitz, MD, MPH
> Clinical Assistant Professor, Department of Family and Preventive Medicine
> Emory University School of Medicine
> Atlanta, GA
> *Drug Safety, Pharmacoeconomics and Pharmacoepidemiology*

Tina Budnitz, MPH
> Senior Advisor for Quality Initiatives
> Society of Hospital Medicine
> Philadelphia, PA
> *Patient Education*
> *Leadership*

Alexander Carbo, MD
> Staff Hospitalist
> Beth Israel Deaconess Medical Center
> Boston, MA
> *Paracentesis*

Niteesh Choudĥry, MD, PhD
> Associate Physician
> Brigham and Women's Hospital
> Boston, MA
> *Diagnostic Decision Making*

Eugene Chu, MD
> Director, Hospital Medicine Program, Denver Health and Hospital Authority
> Assistant Professor of Medicine, University of Colorado Health Sciences Center
> Denver, CO
> *Equitable Allocation of Resources*

Cheryl Clark, MD, SD
> Physician, Internal Medicine
> Brigham and Women's Hospital
> Boston, MA
> *Care of Vulnerable Populations*

Lorenzo DiFrancesco, MD, FACP
> Associate Professor of Medicine
> Emory University School of Medicine
> Atlanta, GA
> *Lumbar Puncture*

Jack Dinh, MD
> Fellow, Division of Gastroenterology
> Robert Wood Johnson Medical School at Camden
> Camden, NJ
> *Professionalism and Medical Ethics*

Brian Donovan, MD
Chief Medical Officer
Global Medical Services, Inc.
Johnson City, TN
Management Practices
Quality Improvement

Daniel Dressler, MD, MSc
Director, Hospital Medicine Services, Emory University Hospital
Assistant Professor of Medicine, Emory University School of Medicine
Atlanta, GA
Transitions of Care

Andrew Epstein, MD
Neurology Resident, Department of Neurology
University of Rochester School of Medicine
Rochester, NY
Professionalism and Medical Ethics

David Feinbloom, MD
Hospitalist
Beth Israel Deaconess Medical Center
Boston, MA
Cardiac Arrhythmia

Scott Flanders, MD
Associate Professor of Medicine
University of Michigan Health System
Ann Arbor, MI
Community-Acquired Pneumonia

Shaun Frost, MD, FACP
Assistant Professor of Medicine
HealthPartners Medical Group and Clinics, University of Minnesota Medical School
St Paul, MN
Perioperative Medicine

Jeffrey Genato, MD
Hospitalist
Hospital Medicine Consultants
Frisic, TX
Vascular Access

Craig Gordon, MD
Instructor
Beth Israel Deaconess Medical Center
Boston, MA
Paracentesis

Adrienne Green, MD
Associate Clinical Professor of Medicine
University of California, San Francisco
San Francisco, CA
Care of the Elderly Patient
Delirium and Dementia

Mahalakshmi Halasyaman, MD
Associate Chair, Department of Internal Medicine
Saint Joseph Mercy Hospital
Ann Arbor, MI
Quality Improvement

John Halporn, MD
>Director, Hospitalist Service
>Emerson Hospital
>Concord, MA
>*Palliative Care*

Gale Hannigan, PhD, MLS, MPH
>Professor and Director, Informatics for Medical Education
>Texas A&M College of Medicine
>College Station, TX
>*Information Management*

Krista Hirschman, PhD
>Medical Educator
>LeHigh Valley Hospital
>Allentown, PA
>*Hospitalist as Teacher*

Russell Holman, MD
>National Medical Director
>Cogent Healthcare
>Raleigh, NC
>*Leadership*

Eric Howell, MD
>Director of the Zieve Medical Services; Associate Director of the Collaborative Inpatient Medical Service,
>Assistant Professor of Medicine
>Johns Hopkins University
>Baltimore, MD
>*Leadership*

Jeanne Huddleston, MD, FACP
>Program Director, Hospital Medicine Fellowship; Assistant Professor of Medicine
>Mayo Clinic College of Medicine
>Rochester, MN
>*Team Approach & Multidisciplinary Care*

Nurcan Ilksoy, MD
>Assistant Professor of Medicine
>Emory University School of Medicine
>Atlanta, GA
>*Congestive Heart Failure*

Amir Jaffer, MD
>Medical Director, Internal Medicine, Perioperative Assessment Consultation and Treatment (IMPACT) Center;
>Medical Director, the Anticoagulation Clinic
>The Cleveland Clinic
>Cleveland, OH
>*Hospitalist as Consultant*

Panch Jeyakumar, MD
>Pulmonary Intensivist
>Chest and Critical Care Consultants
>Anaheim, CA
>*Chest Radiograph Interpretation*
>*Sepsis Syndrome*

Allen Kachalia, MD
>Hospitalist
>Brigham and Women's Hospital
>Boston, MA
>*Risk Management*

Andrew Karson, MD, MPH
Associate Director, Decision Support and Quality Management Unit
Massachusetts General Hospital
Boston, MA
Chronic Obstructive Pulmonary Disease

Surendra Khera, MD
Assistant Director, Internal Medicine Residency Program
Orlando Regional Medical Center
Orlando, FL
Acute Renal Failure

Jennifer Kleinbart, MD
Assistant Professor of Medicine
Emory University School of Medicine
Atlanta, GA
Acute Coronary Syndrome

Valerie Lang, MD
Assistant Professor of Medicine
University of Rochester School of Medicine
Rochester, NY
Alcohol and Drug Withdrawal

Joseph Li, MD
Director, Hospital Medicine Program
Beth Israel Deaconess Medical Center
Boston, MA
Arthrocentesis

David Likosky, MD
Chief of Staff, Director Stroke Program
Evergreen Hospital
Kirkland, WA
Stroke

Susan Marino, MD
Infection Control Practitioner
Brigham and Women's Hospital
Boston, MA
Prevention of Healthcare Associated Infections and Antimicrobial Resistance

George Mathew, MD
Clinical Assistant Professor
Indiana University School of Medicine
Indianapolis, IN
Cellulitis

Sylvia McKean, MD
Medical Director, Brigham and Women's Faulkner Hospitalist Service
Assistant Professor of Medicine, Harvard Medical School
Boston, MA
Drug Safety, Pharmacoeconomics and Pharmacoepidemiology
Hospitalist as Teacher
Patient Education
Patient Handoff
Venous Thromboembolism

Franklin Michota, MD
Head, Section of Hospital Medicine
The Cleveland Clinic Foundation
Cleveland, OH
Perioperative Medicine

Alec O'Connor, MD

    Assistant Professor of Medicine
    University of Rochester School of Medicine
    Rochester, NY
    Alcohol and Drug Withdrawal

Kevin O'Leary, MD

    Assistant Professor of Medicine, Feinberg School of Medicine
    Associate Division Chief for Inpatient Medicine, Northwestern University
    Chicago, IL
    Urinary Tract Infection

Ganiyu Oshodi, MD

    Cardiology Fellow
    MetroHealth Medical Center, Heart and Vascular Center
    Cleveland, OH
    Electrocardiogram Interpretation

Steve Pantilat, MD, FACP

    Associate Professor of Medicine; UCSF Hospitalist Group
    University of California, San Francisco
    San Francisco, CA
    Palliative Care

Michael Pistoria, DO, FACP

    Associate Program Director, Internal Medicine Program; Medical Director, Hospitalist Services
    Lehigh Valley Hospital, Allentown, PA
    Assistant Professor of Medicine, The Pennsylvania State University College of Medicine
    Hershey, PA
    Diabetes Mellitus

Vijay Rajput, MBBS, MS, FACP

    Co-program Director, Internal Medicine Residency, Robert Wood Johnson Medical School
    Senior Hospitalist, Cooper Health System
    Camden, NJ
    Professionalism and Medical Ethics

William Rifkin, MD

    Assistant Professor of Medicine, Yale University School of Medicine,
    Associate Director, Primary Care Residency Program, Waterbury Hospital
    Waterbury, CT
    Pain Management
    Professionalism and Medical Ethics

Malcolm Robinson, MD

    Director, Metabolic Support Service
    Brigham and Women's Hospital
    Boston, MA
    Nutrition and the Hospitalized Patient

Richard Rohr, MD

    Director, Hospitalist Service
    Milford Hospital
    Milford, CT
    Emergency Procedures
    Patient Safety
    Quality Improvement

David Rosenman, MD

    Senior Associate Consultant, Department of Internal Medicine
    Mayo Clinic
    Rochester, MN
    Team Approach and Multidisciplinary Care

Michael Ruhlen, MD, MHCM, FAAP
  Vice President, Medical Affairs
  Toledo Children's Hospital
  Toledo, OH
  Patient Safety
  Quality Improvement

Bindu Sangani, MD
  Staff Hospitalist
  The Cleveland Clinic Foundation
  Cleveland, OH
  Diabetes Mellitus

Gregory Seymann, MD
  Associate Professor, Division of Hospital Medicine
  University of California, San Diego
  San Diego, CA
  Communication
  Gastrointestinal Bleed

Eric Siegal, MD
  Director, Hospital Medicine Program
  University of Wisconsin
  Madison, WI
  Management Practices

Anjala Tess, MD
  Hospitalist
  Beth Israel Deaconess Medical Center
  Boston, MA
  Cardiac Arrhythmia

Anthony Valeri, MD
  Associate Professor of Clinical Medicine; Director, Hemodialysis
  Columbia University Medical Center
  New York, NY
  Acute Renal Failure

Tosha Wetterneck, MD
  Assistant Professor of Medicine
  University of Wisconsin Hospital
  Madison, WI
  Quality Improvement

Chad Whelan, MD
  Assistant Professor of Medicine
  University of Chicago
  Chicago, IL
  Evidence Based Medicine
  Practice Based Learning and Improvement

Mark Williams, MD, FACP
  Professor of Medicine; Director, Emory Hospital Medicine Unit
  Emory University School of Medicine
  Atlanta, GA
  Leadership

Deborah Yokoe, MD, MPH
  Associate Hospital Epidemiologist, Brigham and Women's Hospital
  Assistant Professor of Medicine, Harvard Medical School
  Boston, MA
  Prevention of Healthcare Associated Infections and Antimicrobial Resistance

INTRODUCTION TO THE CORE COMPETENCIES IN HOSPITAL MEDICINE

Background

Hospital Medicine is emerging as the next generation of the site-defined specialties, following Emergency Medicine and Critical Care Medicine. The Society of Hospital Medicine estimates the need for 20,000-30,000 practicing hospitalists in the next five to ten years. A variety of changes in healthcare delivery system and residency training programs has spurred this development. However, this growth has occurred in the absence of any standards of what knowledge, skills and attitudes a hospitalist must possess to successfully practice Hospital Medicine.

The publication of *The Core Competencies in Hospital Medicine: A Framework for Curriculum Development by the Society of Hospital Medicine* (*The Core Competencies*) represents the first attempt to define the specialty of Hospital Medicine. The Core Competencies culminates approximately four years of thoughtful research, planning, and development. *The Core Competencies* are a result of the contributions of over one hundred hospitalists and other content experts, under the guidance and leadership of the SHM Core Curriculum Task Force and Editorial Board. Task Force members were chosen from university and community hospitals, teaching and non-teaching programs, for- and not-for-profit programs, and from all geographic regions of the United States to ensure broad representation of practicing hospitalists and SHM membership. A companion article to this supplement (Dressler DD, Pistoria MJ, Budnitz TL, McKean SCW, Amin AN. Core competencies in hospital medicine: development and methodology. *J Hosp Med.* 2006;1:48-56) details the project methodology.

Purpose

The Core Competencies provide a framework for professional and curricular development based on a shared understanding of the essential knowledge, skills and attitudes expected of physicians working as hospitalists. *The Core Competencies* document specifically targets directors of continuing medical education (CME), Hospitalist programs and fellowships, residency programs, and medical school internal medicine clerkships. The goal is to standardize the expectations for training and professional development and to facilitate the development of

curricula. The competencies were written to reflect learning outcomes, not convey specific content. They can be used to establish targets for learning outcomes. With these targets in mind, instructors can select content and instructional methods and shape the curricula based on the unique characteristics of the intended learners and learning context. A second companion article to the Core Competencies (McKean SCW, Budnitz TL, Dressler DD, Amin AN, Pistoria MJ. How to use The Core Competencies in Hospital Medicine: A Framework for Curriculum Development. *J Hosp Med.* 2006;1:57-67) details how the competencies can be utilized to develop training and curricula to solve specific problems within an institution.

Organization Structure

The Core Competencies comprise three sections—Clinical Conditions, Procedures and Healthcare Systems. Within each section, individual chapters present competencies as three domains of educational outcomes: the Cognitive domain (Knowledge), the Psychomotor domain (Skills), and the Affective domain (Attitudes). The competencies have been carefully crafted as learning outcomes to indicate a specific, measurable level of proficiency that should be expected. Each chapter of the Clinical Conditions and Procedures sections also includes a Systems Organization and Improvement subsection. Outcome statements in this subsection possess attributes of each domain and indicate how the role of hospitalists should evolve. These outcome statements also acknowledge the current variance of responsibilities related to leading, coordinating or participating in the assessment, development or implementation of system improvements. More than any particular knowledge or skill, this systems approach distinguishes a hospitalist from other clinicians practicing in the hospital.

Conclusion

The educational strategy of the Society of Hospital Medicine was to stress the key concepts in hospital medicine in this first edition that would provide a framework for the development of timely, context-specific training and curricula to meet the evolving needs of practicing hospitalists. Therefore, the Task Force selected to include the most commonly encountered clinical conditions, procedures, and healthcare systems that are central to the practice of Hospital Medicine today. We anticipate that future editions will build upon *The Core Competencies* with additional chapters and revisions to reflect feedback from its users, formal evaluation of its application and advances in the field of hospital medicine.

It is our goal that *The Core Competencies in Hospital Medicine* serve as a valuable resource. For the practicing hospitalist, it should aid the refinement of skills and assist in institutional program development. For residency program directors and clerkship directors, the chapters can function as a guide in curriculum development for inpatient medicine rotations or in meeting some of the Accreditation Council on Graduate Medical Education's Outcomes Project. Lastly, for those developing continuing medical education programs, *The Core Competencies* should serve as an outline around which educational programs can be developed.

The Core Curriculum Task Force Editorial Board

Michael J. Pistoria, DO, FACP (Chair)
Alpesh N. Amin, MD, MBA, FACP
Daniel D. Dressler, MD, MSc
Sylvia C. W. McKean, MD
Tina L. Budnitz, MPH

Section 1:   **CLINICAL CONDITIONS**

1.1   Acute Coronary Syndrome
1.2   Acute Renal Failure
1.3   Alcohol and Drug Withdrawal
1.4   Asthma
1.5   Cardiac Arrhythmia
1.6   Cellulitis
1.7   Chronic Obstructive Pulmonary Disease
1.8   Community-Acquired Pneumonia
1.9   Congestive Heart Failure
1.10   Delirium and Dementia
1.11   Diabetes Mellitus
1.12   Gastrointestinal Bleed
1.13   Hospital-Acquired Pneumonia
1.14   Pain Management
1.15   Perioperative Medicine
1.16   Sepsis Syndrome
1.17   Stroke
1.18   Urinary Tract Infection
1.19   Venous Thromboembolism

ACUTE CORONARY SYNDROME

Acute coronary syndrome (ACS) defines a spectrum of ischemic heart disease that may include non-ST-segment elevation myocardial infarction (NSTEMI) and ST-elevation myocardial infarction (STEMI). The American Heart Association (AHA) estimates that 942,000 people with ACS were discharged from acute care hospitals in 2002. This number increased to approximately 1.7 million when including secondary discharge diagnoses. According to the AHA, an estimated $142 billion will be spent on the treatment of heart disease in 2005. Hospitalists diagnose, risk stratify, and initiate early management of patients with ACS. Hospitalists provide leadership for multidisciplinary teams that optimize the quality of inpatient care, maximize opportunities for patient education, and efficiently utilize resources. In addition, hospitalists initiate secondary preventive measures, which increase compliance with outpatient medical regimens.

KNOWLEDGE

Hospitalists should be able to:
- Define and differentiate ACS without enzyme leak, NSTEMI and STEMI.
- Describe the variable clinical presentations of patients with unstable angina and acute myocardial infarction.
- Distinguish ACS from other cardiac and non-cardiac conditions that may mimic this disease process.
- Describe how cardiac biomarkers are used in the diagnosis of ACS, including timing of testing, and the effects of renal disease and other co-morbidities.
- Describe the role of noninvasive cardiac tests.
- Explain indications for and risks associated with cardiac catheterization.
- List the major and minor risk factors predisposing patients to coronary artery disease.
- Explain the value and use of validated risk stratification tools.
- Explain indications for hospitalization of patients with chest pain.
- Explain indications and contraindications for thrombolytic therapy.
- Explain indications, contraindications and mechanisms of action of pharmacologic agents used to treat ACS.
- Describe factors that indicate the need for early invasive interventions, including angiography, stenting and/or coronary artery bypass grafting.
- Identify clinical, laboratory and imaging studies that indicate severity of disease.
- Explain goals for hospital discharge, including specific measures of clinical stability for safe care transition.

SKILLS

Hospitalists should be able to:
- Elicit a thorough and relevant history with emphasis on presenting symptoms and patient risk factors for coronary artery disease (CAD).
- Conduct a physical examination with emphasis on the cardiovascular and pulmonary systems, and recognize clinical signs of ACS and disease severity.
- Diagnose ACS through interpretation of expedited testing including history, physical examination, electrocardiogram, chest radiograph, and biomarkers.
- Perform early risk stratification using validated risk stratification tools.
- Synthesize results of history, physical examination, EKG, laboratory and imaging studies, and risk stratification tools to determine therapeutic options, formulate an evidence-based treatment plan, and determine level of care required.
- Identify patients who may benefit from thrombolytic therapy and/or early revascularization.
- Appreciate and treat patient chest pain, anxiety and other discomfort.
- Recognize symptoms and signs of decompensation and initiate immediate indicated therapies.
- Anticipate and address factors that may complicate ACS or its management, which may include inadequate response to therapies, cardiopulmonary compromise, or bleeding.
- Assess patients with suspected ACS in a timely manner, identify the level of care required, and manage or co-manage the patient with the primary requesting service.

ATTITUDES

Hospitalists should be able to:
- Communicate with patients and families to explain the history and prognosis of their cardiac disease.
- Communicate with patients and families to explain goals of care plan, discharge instructions, and management after release from the hospital.
- Communicate with patients and families to explain tests and procedures, and the use and potential side effects of pharmacologic agents.
- Communicate with patients and families to explain tests and procedures and their indications, and to obtain informed consent.
- Recognize indications for early specialty consultation, which may include cardiology and cardiothoracic surgery.
- Initiate secondary prevention measures prior to discharge, which may include smoking cessation, dietary modification, and evidence based medical therapies.
- Employ a multidisciplinary approach, which may include nursing, nutrition, rehabilitation and social services in the care of patients with ACS that begins at admission and continues through all care transitions.
- Communicate to outpatient providers the notable events of the hospitalization and post-discharge needs, including outpatient cardiac rehabilitation.
- Provide and coordinate resources to patients to ensure safe transition from the hospital to arranged follow-up care.
- Utilize evidence based recommendations and protocols and risk stratification tools for the treatment of ACS.

SYSTEM ORGANIZATION AND IMPROVEMENT

To improve efficiency and quality within their organizations, Hospitalists should:
- Lead, coordinate or participate in efforts to develop protocols to rapidly identify patients with ACS and minimize time to intervention.
- Lead, coordinate or participate in efforts between institutions to develop protocols for the rapid identification and transfer of patients with ACS to appropriate facilities.
- Implement systems to ensure hospital-wide adherence to national standards, and document those measures as specified by recognized organizations (JCAHO, AHA/ACC, AHRQ or others).
- Lead, coordinate or participate in multidisciplinary initiatives to promote patient safety and optimize resource utilization, which may include ACS and chest pain order sets.
- Lead efforts to educate staff on the importance of smoking cessation counseling and other prevention measures.
- Integrate outcomes research, institution-specific laboratory policies, and hospital formulary to create indicated and cost-effective diagnostic and management strategies for patients with ACS.

ACUTE RENAL FAILURE

Acute renal failure (ARF) is defined as a decline in renal function over a period of hours or days, which results in an inability to maintain electrolyte homeostasis and an accumulation of nitrogenous waste products. ARF can be a presenting manifestation of a serious illness requiring hospitalization, or occur as a complication of illness or treatment in a hospitalized patient. The Healthcare Cost and Utilization Project (HCUP) estimates 141,000 discharges for ARF in 2002, with mean charges of almost $22,000 per patient. The mean length of stay was 6.7 days for these patients, with an in-hospital mortality of 10.3%. Hospitalists can advocate and initiate prevention strategies to reduce the incidence of ARF. Hospitalists may also facilitate expeditious evaluation and management of ARF to improve patient outcomes, optimize resource utilization and reduce length of stay.

KNOWLEDGE

Hospitalists should be able to:
- Define the clinical significance of pre-renal failure, intrinsic renal disease, and post-renal failure.
- Describe the symptoms and signs of pre-renal failure, intrinsic renal failure, and post-renal failure.
- Distinguish the causes of pre-renal failure, intrinsic renal failure, and post-renal failure.
- Identify common electrolyte abnormalities that occur with acute renal failure, and institute corrective therapy.
- Describe the indicated tests required to evaluate ARF.
- Calculate estimated creatinine clearance for adjustment of medication dosage when indicated.
- Identify patients at risk for ARF and institute preventive measures, which may include intravenous fluid and acetylcysteine in patients receiving radiocontrast media.
- Identify hospitalized patients at risk for ARF and institute preventive measures.
- Explain indications, contraindications and mechanisms of action of pharmacologic agents used to treat ARF.
- Describe indications for acute hemodialysis.
- Identify clinical, laboratory and imaging studies that indicate severity of disease.
- Explain goals for hospital discharge, including specific measures of clinical stability for safe care transition.

SKILLS

Hospitalists should be able to:
- Elicit a thorough and relevant history and review the medical record for factors predisposing or contributing to the development of ARF.
- Review all drug use including prescription and over-the-counter medications, herbal remedies, nutritional supplements, and illicit drugs.
- Perform a physical examination to assess volume status and to identify underlying co-morbid states that may result in ARF.
- Order and interpret indicated diagnostic studies that may include urinalysis and microscopic sediment analysis, urinary diagnostic indices, urinary protein excretion, serologic evaluation, and renal imaging.
- Avoid use of radiographic contrast agents and order non-ionic agents when available.
- Identify patients who may benefit from early hemodialysis.
- Determine or coordinate appropriate nutritional and metabolic interventions.
- Formulate a treatment plan tailored to the individual patient, which may include fluid management, pharmacologic agents and dosing, nutritional recommendations, and patient compliance.
- Identify and treat factors that may complicate the management of ARF, including extremes of blood pressure and underlying infections.
- Adjust medications according to estimated renal function and route of excretion.
- Avoid use of nephrotoxic agents in ARF. If nephrotoxic agents are required, closely monitor drug levels and renal function.
- Assess patients with suspected ARF in a timely manner, and manage or co-manage the patient with the primary requesting service.

ATTITUDES

Hospitalists should be able to:
- Communicate with patients and families to explain the history and prognosis of ARF.
- Communicate with patients and families to explain goals of care plan, discharge instructions and management after release from hospital.
- Communicate with patients and families to explain tests and procedures, and the use and potential side effects of pharmacologic agents.
- Communicate with patients and families to explain tests and procedures and their indications, and to obtain informed consent.
- Recognize indications for specialty consultation, which may include nephrology or urology.
- Initiate prevention measures including dietary modification and renal dosing of medications.
- Employ a multidisciplinary approach, which may include nursing, nutrition and pharmacy services in the care of patients with ARF that begins at admission and continues through all care transitions.
- Document treatment plan and provide clear discharge instructions for post-discharge physicians.
- Facilitate discharge planning early during hospitalization, including providing the patient with contact information for follow-up care.
- Utilize evidence based recommendations and protocols and risk stratification tools for the treatment of ARF.

SYSTEM ORGANIZATION AND IMPROVEMENT

To improve efficiency and quality within their organizations, Hospitalists should:
- Advocate establishing and supporting initiatives that have been shown to reduce incidence of iatrogenic ARF.
- Lead, coordinate or participate in multidisciplinary teams, which may include nephrology, nursing, pharmacy and nutrition services, to improve processes that facilitate early identification of ARF, early discharge planning, and improved patient outcomes.
- Lead, coordinate or participate in multidisciplinary initiatives to promote patient safety and optimize management strategies for ARF.

ALCOHOL AND DRUG WITHDRAWAL

Alcohol and drug withdrawal is a set of signs and symptoms that develop in association with a sudden cessation or taper in alcohol intake or use of prescription (particularly narcotic medications), over-the-counter (OTC), or illicit drugs. Withdrawal may occur prior to hospitalization or during the course of hospitalization. The Healthcare Cost and Utilization Project (HCUP) estimates 195,000 discharges for alcohol/drug abuse or dependency in 2002. These patients were hospitalized for a mean of 3.9 days with mean charges of $7,266 per patient. Hospitalists can lead their institutions in evidence based treatment protocols that improve care, reduce costs and length of stay, and facilitate better overall outcomes in patients with substance related withdrawal syndromes.

KNOWLEDGE

Hospitalists should be able to:
- Describe the effects of drug and alcohol withdrawal on medical illness and the effects of medical illness on substance withdrawal.
- Recognize the complications from substance use and dependency.
- Distinguish alcohol or drug withdrawal from other causes of delirium.
- Describe the indicated tests required to evaluate alcohol or drug withdrawal.
- Identify patients at increased risk for drug and alcohol withdrawal using current diagnostic criteria for withdrawal.
- Explain indications, contraindications and mechanisms of action of pharmacologic agents used to treat acute alcohol and drug withdrawal.
- Identify local trends in illicit drug use.
- Determine the best setting within the hospital to initiate, monitor, evaluate and treat patients with drug or alcohol withdrawal.
- Explain patient characteristics that on admission portend poor prognosis.
- Explain goals for hospital discharge, including specific measures of clinical stability for safe care transition.

SKILLS

Hospitalists should be able to:
- Elicit a thorough and relevant history, with emphasis on substance use.
- Recognize the symptoms and signs of alcohol and drug withdrawal, including prescription and OTC drugs.
- Differentiate delirium tremens from other alcohol withdrawal syndromes.
- Assess for common co-morbidities in patients with a history of alcohol and drug use.
- Perform a rapid, efficient and targeted physical examination to assess alcohol or drug withdrawal and determine life-threatening co-morbidities.
- Apply DSM-IV Diagnostic Criteria for Alcohol Withdrawal.
- Formulate a treatment plan, tailored to the individual patient, which may include appropriate pharmacologic agents and dosing, route of administration, and nutritional supplementation.
- Integrate existing literature and federal regulations into the management of patients with opioid withdrawal syndromes. For patients who are undergoing existing treatment for opioid dependency, communicate with outpatient treatment centers and integrate dosing regimens into care management.
- Manage withdrawal syndromes in patients with concomitant medical or surgical issues.
- Determine need for the use of restraints to ensure patient safety.
- Reassure, reorient, and frequently monitor the patient in a calm environment.
- Assess patients with suspected alcohol or drug withdrawal in a timely manner, identify the level of care required, and manage or co-manage the patient with the primary requesting service.

ATTITUDES

Hospitalists should be able to:

- Use the acute hospitalization as an opportunity to counsel patients about abstinence, recovery and the medical risks of drug and alcohol use.
- Communicate with patients and families to explain goals of care plan, discharge instructions and management after release from hospital.
- Appreciate the indications for specialty consultations.
- Initiate prevention measures prior to discharge, including alcohol and drug cessation measures.
- Manage the hospitalized patient with substance use in a non-judgmental manner.
- Employ a multidisciplinary approach, which may include psychiatry, pharmacy, nursing and social services, in the treatment of patients with substance use or dependency.
- Establish and maintain an open dialogue with patients and families regarding care goals and limitations.
- Appreciate and document the value of appropriate treatment in reducing mortality, duration of delirium, time required to control agitation, adequate control of delirium, treatment of complications, and cost.
- Facilitate discharge planning early in the hospitalization, including communicating with the primary care provider and presenting the patient with contact information for follow-up care, support and rehabilitation.
- Utilize evidence based national recommendations to guide diagnosis, monitoring and treatment of withdrawal symptoms.

SYSTEM ORGANIZATION AND IMPROVEMENT

To improve efficiency and quality within their organizations, Hospitalists should:

- Lead, coordinate or participate in the development and promotion of guidelines and/or pathways that facilitate efficient and timely evaluation and treatment of patients with alcohol and drug withdrawal.
- Promote the development and use of evidence based guidelines and protocols for the treatment of withdrawal syndromes.
- Advocate for hospital resources to improve the care of patients with substance withdrawal, and the environment in which the care is delivered.
- Lead, coordinate or participate in multidisciplinary teams, which may include psychiatry, to improve patient safety and management strategies for patients with substance abuse.

ASTHMA

Asthma involves bronchospasm with reversible airflow limitation and an abnormal airway inflammatory response. The Healthcare Cost and Utilization Project (HCUP) estimates 130,000 hospital discharges for asthma in 2002. The mean length-of-stay was 2.8 days, with mean charges of $8,000 per patient. When viewed as part of the Diagnosis Related Group (DRG) for Chronic Obstructive Pulmonary Disease, the data is slightly different. These patients accounted for 85,000 discharges with mean charges of almost $14,000 per patient. The mean length-of-stay was 4.6 days in this group, with an in-hospital mortality of 0.6%. Hospitalists use evidence based approaches to optimize care of patients with asthma exacerbation. Hospitalists lead multidisciplinary teams to develop institutional guidelines or care pathways to improve efficiency and quality of care and to reduce readmission rates.

KNOWLEDGE

Hospitalists should be able to:
- Define asthma and describe the pathophysiologic processes that lead to reversible airway obstruction and inflammation.
- Identify precipitants of asthma exacerbation.
- Recognize and differentiate the clinical presentation of asthma exacerbation from other acute respiratory and non-respiratory syndromes.
- Describe the role of diagnostic testing, including peak flow monitoring, used for evaluation of asthma exacerbation.
- Describe evidence based therapies for the treatment of asthma exacerbations, which may include bronchodilators, systemic corticosteroids, and oxygen.
- Explain indications, contraindications and mechanisms of action of pharmacologic agents used to treat asthma.
- Explain the indications for invasive ventilatory support.
- List the risk factors for disease severity and death from asthma.
- Explain goals for hospital discharge, including specific measures of clinical stability for safe care transition.

SKILLS

Hospitalists should be able to:
- Elicit a focused history to identify triggers of asthma and symptoms consistent with asthma exacerbation.
- Perform a targeted physical examination to elicit signs consistent with asthma exacerbation, differentiate findings from other mimicking conditions, and assess severity of illness.
- Select and interpret appropriate diagnostic studies to evaluate severity of asthma exacerbation.
- Recognize impending respiratory failure and coordinate intubation when indicated.
- Prescribe appropriate evidence based pharmacologic therapies during asthma exacerbation, using the most appropriate route, dose, frequency and duration of treatment.

ATTITUDES

Hospitalists should be able to:
- Communicate with patients and families to explain the natural history and prognosis of asthma.
- Communicate with patients and families to explain the goals of care plan, including clinical stability criteria, the importance of prevention measures such as smoking cessation and modification of environmental exposures, and required follow-up care.
- Communicate with patients and families to explain discharge medications, potential side effects, duration of therapy and dosing, and taper schedule.
- Ensure that prior to discharge, patients receive training of proper inhaler and peak flow techniques.
- Differentiate for patients and families the indications and appropriate use of daily use inhalers and rescue inhalers for asthmatic control.
- Communicate with patients and families to explain symptoms and signs that should prompt emergent medical management.
- Recognize indications for specialty consultation, including pulmonary and allergy medicine.
- Promote prevention strategies including smoking cessation and indicated vaccinations.

- Employ a multidisciplinary approach, which may include pulmonary medicine, respiratory therapy, nursing and social services, to the care of patients with asthma exacerbation.
- Collaborate with primary care physicians and emergency physicians in making the admission decision.
- Document treatment plan and discharge instructions, and communicate with the outpatient clinician responsible for follow-up.
- Provide and coordinate resources for patients to ensure safe transition from the hospital to arranged follow-up care.
- Utilize evidence based recommendations for the treatment of patients with asthma exacerbations.

SYSTEM ORGANIZATION AND IMPROVEMENT

To improve efficiency and quality within their organizations, Hospitalists should:
- Develop educational modules, order sets, and/or pathways that facilitate use of evidence based strategies for asthma exacerbation in the emergency department and the hospital, with goals of improving outcomes, decreasing length of stay, and reducing re-hospitalization rates.
- Lead efforts to educate staff on the importance of smoking cessation counseling and other prevention measures.
- Lead, coordinate or participate in multidisciplinary initiatives, which may include collaborative efforts with pulmonologists, to promote patient safety and optimize cost-effective diagnostic and management strategies for patients with asthma.

CARDIAC ARRHYTHMIA

Cardiac arrhythmias are an abnormal heart rate or rhythm. The American Heart Association (AHA) states that in 2002, cardiac arrhythmias were associated with 480,400 deaths and 858,000 hospital discharges. Medical reimbursements for arrhythmia-related diagnoses were $2.2 billion or $6,041 per discharge in 2003. Many arrhythmias may lead to hospitalization or may result as a complication during hospitalization. Hospitalists identify and treat all types of arrhythmias, coordinate specialty and primary care resources, and guide patients safely and cost effectively through the acute hospitalization and back into the outpatient setting.

KNOWLEDGE

Hospitalists should be able to:
- Identify and differentiate the clinical presentation of common arrhythmias.
- Distinguish the causes of atrial and ventricular arrhythmias.
- Describe the indicated tests required to evaluate arrhythmias.
- Explain how medications, metabolic abnormalities and medical co-morbidities may precipitate various arrhythmias.
- Explain indications, contraindications and mechanisms of action of pharmacologic agents used to treat cardiac arrhythmia.
- Risk stratify patients with arrhythmias and determine the level of care required.
- Describe the management goals and options for patients hospitalized with arrhythmia.
- Identify the patient characteristics and co-morbid conditions that predict outcome.
- Explain goals for hospital discharge, including specific measures of clinical stability for safe care transition.

SKILLS

Hospitalists should be able to:
- Elicit a thorough history, including medication, family and social history.
- Perform a directed physical examination with special emphasis on identifying signs associated with hemodynamic stability, tissue perfusion, and occult cardiac and vascular disease.
- Order and interpret EKGs, rhythm monitoring, and telemetry to determine indicated management plan.
- Identify specific arrhythmias by utilizing 12-lead electrocardiogram (EKG) and rhythm strip, and continuous telemetry monitoring.
- Formulate patient-specific, evidence based care plans incorporating diagnostic findings, prognosis and patient characteristics.
- Develop patient-specific care plans that may include rate controlling interventions, cardioversion, defibrillation, or implantable medical devices.
- Utilize telemetry resources for identification of malignant rhythms in patients who require potentially arrhythmegenic interventions or patients who are otherwise at high risk for malignant arrhythmias.
- Limit the use of telemetry resources in patients with chronic stable arrhythmias.
- Quickly recognize high-risk arrhythmias that require urgent intervention, and implement emergency protocols as indicated.
- Assess patients with arrhythmias in a timely manner, identify the level of care required, and manage or co-manage the patient with the primary requesting service.

ATTITUDE

Hospitalists should be able to:
- Communicate with patients and families to explain the history and prognosis of cardiac arrhythmia.
- Communicate with patients and families to explain goals of care plan, discharge instructions and management after release from hospital.
- Communicate with patients and families to explain drug interactions for anti-arrhythmic drugs, and the importance of strict adherence to medication regimens and laboratory monitoring.
- Communicate with patients and families to explain tests and procedures and their indications, and to obtain informed consent.

- Recognize specific arrhythmias or effects of arrhythmias that require early specialty consultation and procedural interventions.
- Employ a multidisciplinary approach, which may include primary care, cardiology, nursing and social services, to develop a care plan for patients with cardiac arrhythmias that begins at admission and continues through all care transitions.
- Acknowledge and ameliorate patient discomfort from uncontrolled arrhythmias and electrical cardioversion therapies.
- Inform receiving physician of pending tests and determine who is responsible for checking results.
- Employ multidisciplinary teams to facilitate discharge planning and communicate to outpatient providers the diagnosis of the arrhythmia, the care plan that occurred in the hospital, and post-discharge needs.
- Utilize evidence based recommendations to guide diagnosis, monitoring and treatment of cardiac arrhythmias.

SYSTEM ORGANIZATION AND IMPROVEMENT

To improve efficiency and quality within their organizations, Hospitalists should:
- Lead, coordinate or participate in multidisciplinary teams to develop patient care guidelines and/or pathways based on peer reviewed outcomes research, patient/physician satisfaction, and cost.
- Implement systems to ensure hospital-wide adherence to national standards and document those measures as specified by recognized organizations (JCAHO, AHA, ACC, AHRQ or others).
- Lead, coordinate or participate in quality improvement initiates to promote early identification of arrhythmias, reduce preventable complications, and promote appropriate use of telemetry resources.

CELLULITIS

Cellulitis is a bacterial infection of the skin and subcutaneous tissues. The Healthcare Cost and Utilization Project (HCUP) states there were approximately 340,000 hospital discharges in 2002 with a Diagnosis Related Group (DRG) for Cellulitis. Patients with cellulitis with complications and co-morbidities had a mean length-of-stay of 5.3 days with an in-hospital mortality of 0.8%. The mean charges for these patients were $13,000. The figures were slightly improved for uncomplicated cellulitis, as the mean length-of-stay dropped to 3.6 days and total charges decreased to $8,000 per patient. Hospitalists can provide leadership to standardize care delivery, improve discharge planning, and promptly identify and address severe cases of cellulitis that require further intervention.

KNOWLEDGE

Hospitalists should be able to:
- Describe the clinical presentation of cellulitis and compare routine and complicated cellulitis.
- Differentiate cellulitis from chronic venous stasis and other conditions that may mimic cellulitis and discuss the accuracy of signs/symptoms in patients admitted with cellulitis.
- Describe the indicated tests required to evaluate cellulitis.
- Relate cellulitis with certain host exposures (including pseudomonas with hot tub exposure, streptococci and venous harvest site cellulitis, and aeromonas with fresh or brackish water).
- Identify patients with co-morbidities (such as the immunocompromised patient, and those with chronic venous and lymphatic problems) and extremes of age (the elderly and the very young) who are at increased risk for a complicated course of cellulitis.
- Differentiate empiric antibiotic regimens for uncomplicated and complicated types of cellulitis.
- Explain indications for inpatient admission.
- Describe the prognostic indicators, including patient co-morbidities, for complicated and uncomplicated cellulitis.
- Explain goals for hospital discharge, including specific measures of clinical stability for safe care transition.

SKILLS

Hospitalists should be able to:
- Elicit a focused history to identify precipitating causes of cellulitis and co-morbid conditions that may impact clinical management.
- Accurately identify and document cellulitis borders and signs of complications, which may include crepitis and abscess.
- Determine and interpret an appropriate and cost-effective initial diagnostic evaluation of cellulitis including laboratory and radiological studies.
- Initiate empiric antibiotic treatment of cellulitis based on host exposures, predisposing underlying systemic illness, history and physical examination, presumptive bacterial pathogens, and evidence based recommendations.
- Treat co-existing fungal infection, edema, and other conditions that may exacerbate cellulitis.
- Formulate a subsequent treatment plan that includes narrowing antibiotic therapies based on available culture data and patient response to treatment.
- Determine appropriate timing for transition from intravenous to oral therapy.
- Assess patients with cellulitis in a timely manner, and manage or co-manage the patient with the primary requesting service.

ATTITUDES

Hospitalists should be able to:
- Communicate with patients and families to explain the history and prognosis of cellulitis.
- Communicate with patients and families to explain goals of care plan, discharge instructions, and management after release from hospital.
- Communicate with patients and families to explain tests and procedures and their indications, and obtain informed consent.
- Recognize the need for early specialty consultation in cases with complications, misdiagnosis, or lack of response to therapy.

- Initiate prevention measures for recurrent cellulites, prior to discharge.
- Employ a multidisciplinary approach to the care of patients with cellulitis that begins at admission and continues through discharge.
- Communicate to outpatient providers the notable events of the hospitalization and anticipated post-discharge needs.
- Consider cost effectiveness (including formulary availability), and ease of conversion to outpatient treatment when choosing among therapeutic options.
- Employ multidisciplinary teams to facilitate discharge planning.
- Utilize evidence based recommendations to guide diagnosis, monitoring and treatment of cellulitis.

SYSTEM ORGANIZATIONS AND IMPROVEMENT

To improve efficiency and quality within their organizations, Hospitalists should:
- Implement systems to ensure hospital-wide adherence to national standards, and document those measures as specified by recognized organizations.
- Lead, coordinate or participate in multidisciplinary initiatives, which may include collaboration with infectious disease physicians, to promote patient safety and optimize cost-effective diagnostic and management strategies for patients with cellulitis.

CHRONIC OBSTRUCTIVE PULMONARY DISEASE

Chronic obstructive pulmonary disease (COPD) involves progressive pulmonary airflow limitation that is not completely reversible, and is associated with an abnormal airway inflammatory response. COPD affects over 11 million Americans and is the fourth most common cause of death in the United States and Canada. COPD exacerbation is defined as an increase in the usual symptoms of COPD and can often result in hospitalization. The Diagnosis Related Group (DRG) for COPD had 652,000 discharges in 2002, according to the Healthcare Cost and Utilization Project (HCUP). Mean charges for these patients were $13,000 per patient and the mean length-of-stay was 4.7 days with in-hospital mortality of 1.7%. Hospitalists use evidence based approaches to optimize care, and can lead multidisciplinary teams to develop institutional guidelines or care pathways to reduce readmission rates and mortality from COPD exacerbation.

KNOWLEDGE

Hospitalists should be able to:
- Define COPD and describe the pathophysiologic processes that lead to small airway obstruction and alveolar destruction.
- Describe potential precipitants of exacerbation, including infectious and non-infectious etiologies.
- Recognize and differentiate the clinical presentation of COPD exacerbation from other acute respiratory and non-respiratory syndromes.
- Describe the role of diagnostic testing used for evaluation of COPD exacerbation.
- Distinguish the medical management of patients with COPD exacerbation from patients with stable COPD.
- Describe the evidence based therapies for treatment of COPD exacerbations, which may include bronchodilators, systemic corticosteroids, oxygen and antibiotics.
- Explain indications, contraindications and mechanisms of action of pharmacologic agents used to treat COPD.
- Describe and differentiate the means of ventilatory support, including the outcome benefits of non-invasive positive pressure ventilation in COPD exacerbation.
- List the indicators of disease severity.
- Explain goals for hospital discharge, including specific measures of clinical stability for safe care transition.

SKILLS

Hospitalists should be able to:
- Elicit a focused history to identify symptoms consistent with COPD exacerbation and etiologic precipitants.
- Perform a targeted physical examination to elicit signs consistent with COPD exacerbation, differentiate it from other mimicking conditions, and assess severity of illness.
- Diagnose patients with COPD exacerbation using history, physical examination, and radiographic data.
- Select and interpret appropriate diagnostic studies to evaluate severity of COPD exacerbation.
- Select patients with COPD exacerbation who would benefit from use of positive pressure ventilation.
- Recognize symptoms, signs and severity of impending respiratory failure and select the indicated evidence based ventilatory approach.
- Prescribe appropriate evidence based pharmacologic therapies during COPD exacerbation, using the most appropriate route, dose, frequency, and duration of treatment.
- Evaluate COPD in perioperative risk assessment, recommend measures to optimize perioperative management of COPD, and manage post-operative complications related to underlying COPD.

ATTITUDES

Hospitalists should be able to:
- Communicate with patients and families to explain the natural history and prognosis of COPD.
- Communicate with patients and families to explain the goals of care plan, including clinical stability criteria, the importance of prevention measures such as smoking cessation, and required follow-up care.
- Communicate with patients and families to explain discharge medications, potential side effects, duration of therapy and dosing, and taper schedule.
- Ensure that prior to discharge patients receive training on proper inhaler techniques and use.

- Recognize indications for specialty consultation, which may include pulmonary medicine.
- Promote prevention strategies including smoking cessation, indicated vaccinations and VTE prophylaxis.
- Recognize the potential risks of supplemental oxygen therapy, including development of hypercarbia in patients with chronic respiratory acidosis.
- Employ a multidisciplinary approach, which may include pulmonary medicine, respiratory therapy, nursing and social services, to the care of patients with COPD exacerbation, beginning at admission and continuing through all care transitions.
- Establish and maintain an open dialogue with patients and/or families regarding care goals and limitations, including palliative care and end-of-life wishes.
- Address resuscitation status early during hospital stay; implement end of life decisions by patients and/or families when indicated or desired.
- Collaborate with primary care physicians and emergency physicians in making the admission decisions.
- Document treatment plan and discharge instructions, and communicate with the outpatient clinician responsible for follow-up.
- Provide and coordinate resources for patients to ensure the safe transition from the hospital to arranged follow-up care.
- Utilize evidence based recommendations for the treatment of patients with COPD exacerbations.

SYSTEM ORGANIZATION AND IMPROVEMENT

To improve efficiency and quality within their organizations, Hospitalists should:
- Develop educational modules, order sets, and/or pathways that facilitate use of evidence based strategies for COPD exacerbation in the emergency department and the hospital, with goals of improving outcomes, decreasing length of stay, and reducing re-hospitalization rates.
- Lead efforts to educate patients and staff on the importance of smoking cessation and other prevention measures.
- Lead, coordinate or participate in multidisciplinary initiatives, which may include collaboration with pulmonologists, to promote patient safety and cost-effective diagnostic and management strategies in the care of patients with COPD.

COMMUNITY-ACQUIRED PNEUMONIA

Community-acquired pneumonia (CAP) is an infection of the lung parenchyma that begins in the community and is diagnosed within 48 hours of admission to the hospital. In the U.S. each year, CAP is the most common infectious cause of death and the sixth leading cause of death overall in the United States. The Healthcare Cost and Utilization Project (HCUP) attributed 831,000 discharges to the Diagnosis Related Group (DRG) for Simple Pneumonia in 2002. These patients were hospitalized for a mean of 5.4 days and had an in-hospital mortality of 4.9%. The mean charges for these patients were $13,000 per patient and the mean length-of-stay was 4.7 days with in-house mortality of 1.7%. Quality indicators have been created around the key processes of care for patients with CAP, and these indicators are used to evaluate performance of states, healthcare organizations, physician groups, and individual physicians. From admission to discharge, hospitalists apply evidence based practice guidelines to the management of CAP and lead initiatives to improve quality of care and reduce practice variability.

KNOWLEDGE

Hospitalists should be able to:
- Define CAP, list the likely etiologies and signs and symptoms, and distinguish from hospital-acquired pneumonia.
- Differentiate CAP from other processes that may mimic CAP or other causes of infiltrates on chest x-ray.
- Describe the indicated tests required to evaluate and treat CAP.
- Explain indications for respiratory isolation.
- Identify patients with co-morbidities (such as the immunocompromised patient and those with diabetes mellitus) and extremes of age (the elderly and very young) who are at risk for a complicated course of CAP.
- Identify specific pathogens that predispose patients to a complicated course of CAP.
- Explain patient specific risk factors and presence of specific organisms that predispose patients to a complicated course of CAP.
- Describe indicated therapeutic modalities for CAP including oxygen therapy, respiratory care modalities and antibiotic selection.
- Predict patient risk for morbidity and mortality from CAP using an evidence based tool such as the Pneumonia Patient Outcomes Research Team (PORT) / Pneumonia Severity Index (PSI) validated risk score.
- Explain goals for hospital discharge, including evidence based measures of clinical stability for safe care transition.

SKILLS

Hospitalists should be able to:
- Elicit a focused history to identify symptoms consistent with CAP and demographic factors that may predispose patients to CAP.
- Perform a targeted physical examination to elicit signs consistent with CAP and differentiate it from other mimicking conditions.
- Select and interpret indicated laboratory, microbiologic and radiological studies to confirm diagnosis of CAP, and risk stratify patients.
- Apply evidence based tools such as the pneumonia severity index, to triage decisions and identify factors that support the need for intensive care unit (ICU) admission.
- Initiate empiric antibiotic selection based on exposure to long term or group care, severity of illness, and evidence based national guidelines, taking into account local resistance patterns.
- Formulate a subsequent treatment plan that includes narrowing antibiotic therapies based on available culture data and patient response to treatment.
- Recognize and address complications of CAP and/or inadequate response to therapy including respiratory failure and emerging parapneumonic effusions.

ATTITUDES

Hospitalists should be able to:

- Communicate with patients and families to explain the history and prognosis of CAP.
- Communicate with patients and families to explain the goals of care plan, including clinical stability criteria, the importance of prevention measures such as smoking cessation, and required follow-up care.
- Communicate with patients and families to explain tests and procedures, and the use and potential side effects of pharmacologic agents.
- Recognize indications for specialty consultation.
- Promote prevention strategies, which may include smoking cessation and indicated vaccinations.
- Collaborate with primary care physicians and emergency physicians in making the admission decision.
- Document treatment plan and discharge instructions, and identify the outpatient clinician responsible for follow-up of pending tests.
- Recognize and address barriers to follow-up care and anticipated post-discharge requirements.
- Utilize evidence based recommendations for the treatment of patients with CAP

SYSTEM ORGANIZATION AND IMPROVEMENT

To improve efficiency and quality within their organizations, Hospitalists should:

- Lead, coordinate or participate in efforts to identify, address and monitor quality indicators for CAP including assessment of oxygenation, obtaining blood cultures prior to administration of antibiotics, prompt administration of antibiotics, and providing indicated vaccinations and smoking cessation education.
- Implement systems to ensure hospital wide adherence to national standards and document those measures as specified by recognized organizations (JCAHO, IDSA, ATS)
- Integrate PORT score / PSI in conjunction with patient specific factors and clinical judgment into the admission decision.
- Lead, coordinate or participate in multidisciplinary initiatives, which may include collaboration with infectious disease and pulmonary specialists, to promote patient safety and cost effective diagnostic and management strategies for patients with CAP.
- Lead efforts to educate staff on the importance of smoking cessation counseling and other prevention measures.

CONGESTIVE HEART FAILURE

Congestive heart failure syndrome (CHF) is characterized by impaired function of the heart resulting in a constellation of symptoms and signs, which may include fatigue, weakness and shortness of breath. The American Heart Association (AHA) reports that CHF affects nearly 5 million people in the United States. CHF accounted for 970,000 hospital discharges in 2002. Medicare paid $3.6 billion for the care of patients with CHF in 1999, or $5,456 per discharge. The estimated direct and indirect cost of CHF in 2005 is $27.9 billion. Despite published guidelines for CHF management, there is significant variation in treatment for hospitalized patients. This variability significantly impacts individual patients, families and hospital systems, and accounts for billions of dollars of the Medicare budget. Hospitalists can lead their institutions in early diagnosis, initiation of evidence based medical therapy, and incorporation of a multidisciplinary approach to heart failure. Hospitalists can also develop strategies to operationalize cost-effective interventions that reduce morbidity, mortality and readmission rates.

KNOWLEDGE

Hospitalists should be able to:
- Explain underlying causes of CHF and precipitating factors leading to exacerbation.
- Differentiate features of systolic and diastolic dysfunction, and explain the common etiologies of each.
- Describe the indicated tests required to evaluate CHF, including assessment of left ventricular function.
- Describe risk factors for the development of CHF in the hospital setting.
- Risk stratify patients admitted with CHF and determine the appropriate level of care.
- Describe goals of inpatient therapy for acute decompensated heart failure including pre-load and after-load reduction, hemodynamic stabilization, and optimization of volume status.
- Describe the role of invasive and noninvasive ventilatory support.
- Explain evidence based therapeutic options for management of acute and chronic CHF and describe contraindications to these therapies.
- Explain indications, contraindications and mechanisms of action of pharmacologic agents used to treat CHF.
- Identify medications and interventions contraindicated in CHF.
- Explain markers of severity of the disease and factors that influence prognosis.
- Explain goals for hospital discharge, including specific measures of clinical stability for safe care transition.

SKILLS

Hospitalists should be able to:
- Elicit a thorough and relevant history and review the medical record to identify symptoms, co-morbidities, medications, and/or social influences contributing to CHF or its exacerbation.
- Review inpatient records to determine iatrogenic influences of CHF.
- Recognize the clinical presentation of heart failure, including features of exacerbation and reliability of signs and symptoms.
- Identify physical findings consistent with CHF.
- Identify signs of low perfusion states and cardiogenic shock.
- Order indicated diagnostic testing to identify precipitating factors of CHF and assess cardiac function.
- Formulate an evidence based treatment plan, tailored to the individual patient, which may include pharmacologic agents and dosing, nutritional recommendations, and patient compliance.
- Recognize symptoms and signs of acute decompensation and initiate immediate indicated therapies.
- Assess patients with suspected heart failure in a timely manner, identify the level of care required, and manage or co-manage the patient with the primary requesting service.

ATTITUDES

Hospitalists should be able to:
- Communicate with patients and families to explain the history and prognosis of CHF.
- Communicate with patients and families to explain the importance of home self-monitoring and adherence to medication regimens, nutritional recommendations, and physical rehabilitation.

- Communicate with patients and families to explain goals of care plan, discharge instructions and management after release from hospital.
- Communicate with patients and families to explain tests and procedures, and the use and potential side effects of pharmacologic agents.
- Recognize indications for early cardiology consultation.
- Recognize indications and qualifications for cardiac transplant evaluation.
- Advocate the importance of behavioral modification to delay the progression of disease and improve quality of life.
- Employ a multidisciplinary approach to the care of patients with CHF that begins at admission and continues through all care transitions.
- Recognize the importance of palliative care in the treatment of patients with chronic CHF.
- Responsibly address and respect end of life care wishes for patients with end-stage CHF.
- Communicate to outpatient providers the relevant events of the hospitalization and post-discharge needs, including pending tests, and determine who is responsible for checking the results.
- Document treatment plan and provide clear discharge instructions for receiving primary care physician.
- Utilize evidence based recommendations to guide diagnosis, monitoring and treatment of CHF.

SYSTEM ORGANIZATION AND IMPROVEMENT

To improve efficiency and quality within their organizations, Hospitalists should:
- Advocate to hospital administrators to establish and support outpatient CHF teams, which have been shown to reduce readmission rates and possibly morbidity and mortality through outreach to CHF patients.
- Lead, coordinate or participate in multidisciplinary teams, which may include nursing and social services, nutrition, pharmacy, and physical therapy, early in the hospital course to facilitate patient education and discharge planning; improve patient function and outcomes; and advocate patient outreach post-discharge.
- Implement systems to ensure hospital wide adherence to national standards and document those measures as specified by recognized organizations (JCAHO, AHA, ACC, AHRQ or others).
- Lead, coordinate or participate in multidisciplinary initiatives to promote patient safety and optimize resource utilization.
- Lead efforts to educate staff on the importance of smoking cessation counseling and other prevention measures.
- Integrate outcomes research, institution-specific laboratory policies, and hospital formulary to create indicated and cost-effective diagnostic and management strategies for patients with CHF.

DELIRIUM AND DEMENTIA

Delirium is defined as a transient global disorder of cognition. Many factors lead to delirium including baseline vulnerability interacting with precipitants during hospitalization. Delirium affects an estimated 2.3 million hospitalized elders annually, accounting for 17.5 million inpatient days, and leading to more than $4 billion in Medicare costs. It is associated with increased mortality, high rates of functional and cognitive decline, prolonged lengths of stay and high rates of skilled nursing facility placement. The cost of caring for patients with delirium significantly impacts individual patients, families and hospital systems, and accounts for billions of the Medicare budget. Hospitalists lead their institutions in the development of screening and prevention protocols for patients at risk for delirium, and in the promotion of safe approaches to treatment. Hospitalists also develop strategies to operationalize cost-effective delirium prevention programs that will improve outcomes.

Dementia is defined as a progressive decline in cognitive function, eventually limiting daily activities. Dementia is a common co-morbidity in the hospitalized elder. Patients with dementia are at increased risk for delirium, falls, and functional decline during hospitalization. Patients with baseline cognitive impairment have prolonged lengths of stay and complex needs after discharge. Agitation and behavioral symptoms of dementia can exacerbate and be difficult to manage in the hospital setting. Care of the patient with dementia requires that hospitalists engage in a multidisciplinary approach to inpatient and transitional care. Hospitalists may also become involved in hospital quality and safety initiatives that pertain to areas such as restraint use and fall prevention.

KNOWLEDGE

Hospitalists should be able to:
- Define delirium and dementia.
- Distinguish the causes of delirium.
- Describe the indicated tests required to evaluate delirium and dementia.
- Recognize innate and environmental/iatrogenic risk factors for the development of delirium in the hospitalized patient.
- Identify medications known to precipitate delirium.
- Explain indications, contraindications and mechanisms of action of pharmacologic agents used to treat delirium and dementia.
- Determine the best setting within the hospital to initiate, monitor, evaluate and treat patients with delirium.
- Describe the poor outcomes related to delirium and dementia in the hospitalized patient.
- Explain goals for hospital discharge, including specific measures of clinical stability for safe care transition.

SKILLS

Hospitalists should be able to:
- Distinguish delirium and dementia from other causes of cognitive impairment, confusion or psychosis.
- Predict a patient's risk for the development of delirium or poor outcomes related to dementia based on initial history and physical examination.
- Screen for delirium using appropriate testing early and repeatedly during the patient's hospital course.
- Perform a screen for dementia using the appropriate testing.
- Apply known patient risk factors to create a care plan for reducing delirium.
- Perform a focused evaluation for the underlying etiology of delirium and institute prompt treatment to lessen the severity of delirium.
- Formulate and lead multidisciplinary teams to develop and implement care plans for patients with delirium or dementia.
- Prescribe appropriate medications and dosing regimens for patients with delirium or dementia.
- Repeatedly assess the need for additional interventions.
- Assess patients with suspected delirium in a timely manner, identify the level of care required, and manage or co-manage the patient with the primary requesting service.

ATTITUDES

Hospitalists should be able to:
- Communicate with patients and families to explain the history and prognosis of delirium or dementia.
- Communicate with patients and families to explain goals of care plan, discharge instructions and management after release from hospital.
- Educate and engage families in the care of elder inpatients.
- Establish goals and boundaries of care with patients and their family.
- Communicate with the families and others with durable powers of attorney to explain tests and procedures and their indications, and to obtain informed consent.
- Recognize the indications for specialty consultations.
- Describe methods for the prevention of delirium.
- Employ a multidisciplinary approach to the care of patients with delirium or dementia that begins at admission and continues through all care transitions.
- Responsibly address and respect end of life care wishes for patients with advanced dementia.
- Realize the multi-faceted impact of delirium or dementia on patients and their families.
- Appreciate and document the value of appropriate treatment in reducing mortality, duration of delirium, time required to control agitation, adequate control of delirium, treatment of complications, and cost.
- Facilitate discharge planning early in the hospitalization, including communicating with the primary care provider, and presenting the patient and family with contact information for follow-up care, support and rehabilitation.
- Utilize evidence based recommendations to guide diagnosis, monitoring and treatment of delirium and its causes.

SYSTEM ORGANIZATION AND IMPROVEMENT

To improve efficiency and quality within their organizations, Hospitalists should:
- Lead multidisciplinary teams to develop early treatment protocols.
- Lead, coordinate or participate in multidisciplinary initiatives to implement screening and prevention protocols for patients at risk for delirium or poor outcomes related to dementia.
- Engage stakeholders in hospital initiatives to improve safety and quality in the care of delirious and demented patients (e.g. provide diversion activities rather than using restraints).
- Lead, coordinate or participate in multidisciplinary initiatives, which may include collaboration with
- geriatricians, to promote patient safety and cost-effective diagnostic and management strategies for elderly patients.

DIABETES MELLITUS

Diabetes mellitus is a disease characterized by abnormal insulin production or disordered glucose metabolism and is a co-morbid condition of many hospitalized patients. Diabetic ketoacidosis (DKA) and hyperglycemia hyperosmolar state (HHS) are extreme presentations of diabetes mellitus that require hospitalization. There were 577,000 hospital discharges for diabetes mellitus in 2002, according to the American Heart Association. The prevalence of physician-diagnosed diabetes mellitus was 13.9 million or 6.7 percent of the United States population. Another 5.9 million Americans are believed to have undiagnosed diabetes mellitus. The Healthcare Cost and Utilization Project (HCUP) reports an average length-of-stay of 4.1 days and mean charges of $11,761 per patient for the Diagnosis Related Group (DRG) for Diabetes Mellitus. The estimated economic cost of diabetes in 2002 was $132 billion, of which $92 billion was direct medical costs. Hospitalists care for diabetic patients and optimize glycemic control in the hospital setting. They stabilize and treat DKA and HHS. The inpatient setting provides an opportunity to institute therapies to slow disease progression, prevent disease complications, and provide diabetic education to improve quality of life and limit complications leading to readmission. Hospitalists use evidence based approaches to optimize care and lead multidisciplinary teams to develop institutional guidelines or care pathways to optimize glycemic control.

KNOWLEDGE

Hospitalists should be able to:
- Define diabetes mellitus and explain the pathophysiologic processes that can lead to hyperglycemia, DKA and HHS.
- Describe the impact of hyperglycemia on immune function and wound healing.
- Describe the effect of DKA and HHS on intravascular volume status, electrolytes and acid-base balance.
- Describe the clinical presentation and laboratory findings of DKA and HHS.
- Describe the indicated tests to evaluate and diagnose DKA and HHS.
- Explain physiologic stressors and medications that adversely impact glycemic control.
- Explain the precipitating factors of DKA and HSS.
- Identify the goals of glycemic control in hospitalized patients in various settings, including critically ill and surgical patients, and cite supporting evidence.
- Explain indications, contraindications and mechanisms of action of pharmacologic agents used to treat diabetes mellitus.
- Explain the rationale of strict glycemic control and its effects on morbidity and mortality in hospitalized patients.
- Recognize factors that indicate severity of disease in patients with DKA or HHS.
- Explain goals for hospital discharge, including specific measures of clinical stability for safe care transition.

SKILLS

Hospitalists should be able to:
- Elicit a thorough and relevant history, and review the medical record to identify symptoms suggestive of acute co-morbid illness that can impact glycemic control.
- Estimate the level of outpatient glycemic control, adherence to medication regimen, and social influences that may impact glycemic control.
- Perform a comprehensive physical examination to identify possible precipitants of hyperglycemia, DKA or HHS.
- Identify precipitating factors for DKA and HHS, including infection, myocardial ischemia, and adherence to medication regimen.
- Select and interpret indicated studies in patients suspected of having DKA or HHS, including electrolytes, beta-hydroxybuterate, urinalysis, venous pH, and electrocardiogram.
- Recognize the indications for managing DKA and HHS in an intensive care unit.
- Select appropriate insulin therapies, initiate fluid resuscitation, and manage the electrolyte disturbances caused by DKA and HHS.
- Adjust medications to achieve optimal glycemic control and minimize side effects.

- Assess caloric and nutritional needs and order appropriate diabetic diet.
- Recognize and address neuropathic pain.
- Anticipate and manage the presence of ongoing metabolic derangements associated with DKA and HHS.
- Develop an individualized diabetic regimen to achieve optimal glycemic control and prevent the development of complications from diabetes mellitus, including during the perioperative period.

ATTITUDES

Hospitalists should be able to:
- Communicate with patients and families to explain the history and prognosis of diabetes mellitus.
- Communicate with patients and families to explain potential long-term complications of diabetes mellitus and prevention strategies, including foot and eye care.
- Communicate with patients and families to explain goals of care plan, discharge instructions and management after release from the hospital.
- Communicate with patients and families to explain the importance of and factors affecting glycemic control, such as adherence to medical regimens and self-monitoring, following dietary and exercise recommendations, and complying with routine follow-up appointments.
- Communicate with patients and families to explain the potential side effects or adverse interactions of diabetes medications, including hypoglycemia.
- Recognize indications for early specialty consultation, which may include endocrinology and nutrition.
- Employ a multidisciplinary approach, which may include nursing, nutrition and social services and a diabetes educator, to the care of patients with diabetes that begins at admission and continues through all care transitions.
- Document treatment plan and discharge instructions, and communicate with the outpatient clinician responsible for follow-up, including the need for continued nutrition and diabetic counseling.
- Facilitate discharge planning early in the admission process.
- Recommend appropriate post-discharge care, which may include endocrinology, ophthalmology, and podiatry.
- Utilize evidence based recommendation in the treatment of inpatients with diabetes mellitus.

SYSTEM ORGANIZATION AND IMPROVEMENT

To improve efficiency and quality within their organizations, Hospitalists should:
- Implement systems to ensure hospital-wide adherence to national standards (American Diabetes Association and others), and document those measures as specified by recognized organizations.
- Lead, coordinate or participate in efforts to develop guidelines and protocols that standardize assessment and aggressive treatment of DKA and HHS.
- Lead, coordinate or participate in efforts to develop guidelines and/or protocols to optimize glycemic control in hospitalized patients, including intensive regimens in critically ill medical and surgical patients.
- Lead, coordinate or participate in multidisciplinary teams, which may include nursing, nutrition and endocrinology, to promote quality and cost-effective diabetes management.

GASTROINTESTINAL BLEED

Gastrointestinal (GI) bleed refers to any bleeding that originates in the GI tract. Bleeding is generally defined as upper (between the mouth and ligament of Treitz) or lower (from the ligament of Treitz to the anus). Healthcare Cost and Utilization Project (HCUP) 2002 data for the Diagnosis Related Group (DRG) for GI Bleed with complications or co-morbidities reveals approximately 409,000 discharges with an in-hospital mortality of 3.0%. The mean length-of-stay for these patients was 4.4 days, with mean charges of $15,000. Hospitalists provide immediate care for these patients, who often require coordination of care across multiple specialties. Hospitalists lead quality improvement initiatives that optimize the efficiency and quality of care for these patients.

KNOWLEDGE

Hospitalists should be able to:
- Explain the multiple potential etiologies or pathophysiologic processes that lead to GI bleeds.
- Describe and differentiate the clinical features and presentations of upper and lower GI bleeds.
- Explain the differential diagnosis for the most common causes of upper and lower GI bleeds.
- Describe the indicated tests required to evaluate GI bleeds.
- Explain the risk factors for upper and lower GI bleeds, and clinical indicators of patients at high risk for complications.
- Explain the factors that may require early aggressive interventions or increase patient risk for recurrent bleeds.
- Risk stratify patients with GI bleeds and determine the level of care required.
- Describe the indications for transfusion therapy in GI bleeds, and explain the various methods of treatment for coagulopathy.
- Compare the advantages and disadvantages of medical, endoscopic, and surgical treatments for patients with upper and lower GI bleeds.
- Explain indications, contraindications and mechanisms of action of pharmacologic agents used to treat GI bleeds.
- Explain patient characteristics that on admission portend poor prognosis.
- Identify clinical, laboratory and imaging studies that indicate severity of disease.
- Explain goals for hospital discharge, including specific measures of clinical stability for safe care transition.

SKILLS

Hospitalists should be able to:
- Elicit a thorough and relevant history, including a directed medication, family and social history.
- Perform a physical examination and identify clinical indicators of upper and lower GI bleeds, and evidence of underlying states, which may include liver disease.
- Recognize physical findings that indicate clinical instability due to acute blood loss, including digital rectal examination, and interpretation of orthostatic blood pressure and pulse measurements.
- Insert a nasogastric tube, perform a gastric lavage, and interpret the results.
- Order and interpret results of appropriate laboratory, imaging, and endoscopic testing.
- Synthesize results of physical examination, laboratory and imaging studies to determine the best management and care plan for the patient.
- Formulate an evidence based treatment plan including nutritional recommendations, pharmacologic agents and dosing, and coordination of endoscopic and surgical interventions tailored to the individual patient.
- Determine frequency for laboratory monitoring and transfusion during hospitalization.
- Assure adequate intravenous access to allow rapid volume and blood product resuscitation.
- Perform rapid hemodynamic resuscitation.
- Recognize and treat signs of clinical decompensation and recurrent bleeding.
- Assess patients with suspected GI bleeds in a timely manner, and manage or co-manage the patient with the primary requesting service.

ATTITUDES

Hospitalists should be able to:
- Communicate with patients and families to explain the disease etiology, prognosis, risk reduction strategies, and symptoms of recurrent GI bleed.
- Communicate with patients and families to explain goals of care plan, discharge instructions and management after release from hospital.
- Communicate with patients and families to explain risks, benefits, and alternatives to transfusion therapy.
- Communicate with patients and families to explain tests and procedures and their indications, and to obtain informed consent.
- Recognize the indications for early specialty consultation, which may include interventional radiology, gastroenterology and surgery.
- Initiate prevention measures including avoidance of NSAIDs, stress ulcer prophylaxis in critically ill patients, dietary modification, and evidence based medical therapies.
- Employ a multidisciplinary approach, which may include nursing, pharmacy and nutrition services, and specialty and referring physicians, to the care of patients with GI bleeds.
- Employ a multidisciplinary approach to the care of patients with GI bleed that begins at admission and continues through all care transitions.
- Establish and maintain an open dialogue with patients and families regarding care goals and limitations, including palliative care and end-of-life wishes.
- Address resuscitation status early during hospital stay; discuss and implement end-of-life decisions by patient or family when indicated or desired.
- Inform receiving physician of pending study results.
- Employ multidisciplinary teams to facilitate discharge planning and communicate to outpatient providers the notable events of the hospitalization and anticipated post-discharge needs.

SYSTEM ORGANIZATION AND IMPROVEMENT

To improve efficiency and quality within their organizations, Hospitalists should:
- Lead, coordinate or participate in the development and promotion of guidelines and/or pathways that facilitate efficient and timely evaluation and treatment of patients with GI bleeds.
- Lead, coordinate or participate in multidisciplinary teams, which may include emergency medicine physicians, gastroenterologists and nurses, to develop quality improvement initiatives that promote early identification of GI bleeds and reduce preventable complications.
- Develop systems that provide timely reports of pending study results to outpatient providers.
- Integrate outcomes research, institution-specific laboratory policies, and hospital formulary to create indicated and cost-effective diagnostic and management strategies for patients with GI bleeds.

HOSPITAL-ACQUIRED PNEUMONIA

Hospital-acquired pneumonia (HAP) is an infection of the lung parenchyma that occurs during the course of hospitalization. HAP is a significant source of morbidity, mortality, and increased resource expenditures. The attributable mortality for HAP is in the 30-50 percent range. The primary risk factor for the development of HAP is mechanical ventilation. The average length of stay for patients with HAP increases by an average of 13 days, with estimated additional costs of $40,000. Hospitalists manage patients with HAP either as an attending physician or as a consultant to patients admitted to other services. Hospitalists can initiate quality improvement strategies at the individual patient level and at the system level to improve patient outcomes and optimize resource utilization.

KNOWLEDGE

Hospitalists should be able to:
- Define hospital-acquired pneumonia (HAP).
- List common organisms associated with HAP.
- Describe local and national resistance patterns for HAP.
- Identify important historical elements, medical record data and physical examination findings consistent with HAP.
- Distinguish the infectious causes of HAP.
- Describe the indicated tests required to evaluate HAP.
- Identify patients at risk for developing HAP.
- Describe the role of mechanical ventilation as a risk factor for the development of HAP.
- Explain the prophylactic measures commonly used to lower the risk of HAP.
- Describe the role of mechanical ventilation as a potential treatment option for HAP.
- Describe infection control practices to prevent the spread of resistant organisms within the hospital.
- Describe potential complications of HAP.
- Explain goals for hospital discharge, including specific measures of clinical stability for safe care transition.

SKILLS

Hospitalists should be able to:
- Elicit a thorough and relevant history, and perform a targeted physical examination for hospital-acquired pneumonia.
- Order and interpret indicated laboratory, microbiologic and radiological studies to confirm diagnosis of hospital acquired pneumonia and determine the etiologic agent.
- Initiate empiric antibiotic regimen based on patient history and underlying co-morbid conditions, likely organisms and local resistance patterns.
- Tailor antibiotic regimens based on microbiologic culture and sensitivity data as soon as available.
- Manage complications, which may include respiratory failure, pleural effusions and empyema.
- Coordinate care for patients requiring mechanical ventilation.
- Identify patients who require thoracentesis, perform or coordinate the procedure, and interpret the results.
- Assess patients with suspected hospital-acquired pneumonia in a timely manner, and manage or co-manage the patient with the primary requesting service.

ATTITUDES

Hospitalists should be able to:
- Communicate with patients and families to explain the etiology, management plan, and potential outcomes of hospital-acquired pneumonia.
- Communicate with patients and families to explain the tests and procedures and their indications, and to obtain informed consent.
- Recognize indications for specialty consultation, which may include infectious disease and/or pulmonary services.
- Employ a multidisciplinary approach, which may include nursing, respiratory therapy, nutrition and pharmacy services, to the care of patients with HAP through all care transitions.

- Recognize steps that can be employed to limit the emergence of antibiotic resistance.
- Document treatment plan and provide clear discharge instructions for post-discharge physicians.
- Recognize implications of HAP on discharge planning.
- Lead multidisciplinary teams to facilitate discharge planning, and communicate to outpatient providers the notable events of the hospitalization and anticipated post-discharge needs.
- Utilize evidence based recommendations and protocols and risk stratification tools for the treatment of HAP.

SYSTEM ORGANIZATION AND IMPROVEMENT

To improve efficiency and quality within their organizations, Hospitalists should:
- Collaborate with local infection control practitioners to reduce the spread of resistant organisms within the institution.
- Lead, coordinate or participate in multidisciplinary initiatives, which may include collaboration with critical care specialists and pulmonologists, to reduce the incidence of hospital-acquired pneumonia in ventilated patients.
- Lead, coordinate or participate in quality improvement initiatives to reduce ventilator days, rates of HAP, and variance in antibiotic use.
- Implement systems to ensure hospital-wide adherence to national standards for empiric antibiotic use, and document those measures as specified by recognized organizations.
- Lead efforts to educate staff on the importance of smoking cessation counseling and other prevention measures.

PAIN MANAGEMENT

Pain, defined by International Association for the Study of Pain (IASP), as "an unpleasant experience associated with actual or potential tissue damage to a person's body", is a very common presenting or accompanying symptom of hospitalized patients. Pain management involves utilizing various modalities to alleviate suffering and restore patient function. Proper assessment and treatment of pain can improve clinical outcomes, discharge planning and patient and family satisfaction. Pain management of inpatients necessitates understanding the various mechanisms that cause pain, properties of analgesic pharmacological and non-pharmacological modalities, as well as the accurate assessment of severity and treatment response. Hospitalists assess and manage patients experiencing pain. This role encompasses empathy, clinical excellence, and understanding of the myriad obstacles, cautions and specific knowledge, skills and attitudes necessary for appropriate pain management. Hospitalists serve as leaders of multidisciplinary teams to develop policies and protocols to improve pain management in their health care system.

KNOWLEDGE

Hospitalists should be able to:
- Describe the mechanisms that cause pain.
- Describe the symptoms and signs of pain.
- Differentiate acute, chronic, somatic, neuropathic, referred and visceral pain syndromes.
- Differentiate tolerance, dependence, addiction and pseudo-addiction.
- Describe the value and limitations of the physical examination and various validated pain intensity assessment scales.
- Explain the relationship between physical, cultural and psychological factors and pain and pain thresholds.
- Discuss the genetic, social, and psychological factors that may contribute to opioid addiction.
- Explain the indications and limitations of non-pharmacological methods of pain control available in the inpatient setting.
- Explain the indications and limitations of non-opioids including acetaminophen, nonsteroidal anti-inflammatory drugs (NSAIDs), and topical agents.
- Explain the indications and limitations of opioid pharmacotherapy.
- Explain the indications and limitations of other analgesics including, tramadol, tricyclic agents and anti-epileptic medications in the treatment of various pain syndromes.
- Describe specific factors that affect dosing regimes, such as drug half-life, renal and hepatic function.
- Establish functional criteria for discharge.

SKILLS

Hospitalists should be able to:
- Elicit a detailed history and description of pain and review the medical record to determine likely source and acuity of pain.
- Review patient pharmacologic and psychosocial history and identify factors contributing to pain or factors that might impact its management.
- Conduct a physical examination to determine the likely source of pain.
- Order and interpret diagnostic studies to determine the source of pain when underlying acute illness is suspected.
- Assess pain severity using validated measurement tools.
- Formulate an initial pain management plan.
- Determine appropriate route, dosing and frequency for pharmacologic agents based on patient-specific factors.
- Reassess pain severity and determine the need for escalating therapy and/or adjuvant therapies.
- Determine equianalgesic dosing for pharmacologic therapy when needed.
- Titrate short and long acting narcotics to desired effect.
- Predict and counteract as needed expected analgesic side effects, including use of reversal and specific agents, especially in elderly.

- Initiate appropriate therapies to prevent and treat constipation when using opioid analgesics.
- Anticipate and manage side effects of pain medications including respiratory depression and sedation, nausea, vomiting and pruritis.
- Assess and communicate need for pain management during medical consultation.

ATTITUDES

Hospitalists should be able to:
- Promote the ethical imperative of frequent pain assessment and adequate control.
- Appreciate that all pain is subjective and acknowledge patients' self-reports of pain.
- Appreciate the value of patient controlled analgesia.
- Discuss with patients and families the goals for pain management strategies and functional status, and set targets for pain control.
- Recognize indications for specialty consultation, which may include pain service, anesthesiology, and physical and rehabilitation medicine.
- Employ a multidisciplinary approach to the assessment and management of patients with pain that begins on admission and continues through all care transitions.
- Educate patients and physicians on the importance of appropriate use of opioids in pain management and explain the rarity of opioid addiction in the setting of appropriate pain management.
- Establish and maintain an open dialogue with patients and families regarding care goals and limitations, which may include palliative care and end-of-life wishes.
- Address resuscitation status early during hospital stay; implement end-of-life decisions by patient and/or family when indicated or desired.
- Document treatment plan and discharge instructions, and communicate with the outpatient clinician responsible for follow-up.
- Provide and coordinate resources to patients to ensure safe transition from the hospital to arranged follow-up care.
- Utilize evidence based recommendations, including the World Health Organization (WHO) step approach to pain management.

SYSTEM ORGANIZATION AND IMPROVEMENT

To improve efficiency and quality within their organizations, Hospitalists should:
- Lead, coordinate, or participate in efforts to develop educational modules, order sets, and/or pathways that facilitate effective pain management in the hospital setting, with goals of improving outcomes and patient satisfaction, decreasing length of stay, and reducing re-hospitalization rates.
- Lead, coordinate or participate in efforts to measure quality of inpatient pain control and operationalize system improvements and reduction of barriers to adequate pain control
- Lead, coordinate or participate in efforts to establish or support existing multidisciplinary pain control teams.

PERIOPERATIVE MEDICINE

Perioperative medicine refers to the medical evaluation and management of patients before, during and after surgical intervention. In the United States, over 44 million patients undergo non-cardiac surgery each year. The annual cost of perioperative cardiovascular morbidity is more than $20 billion. Hospitalists perform general medical consultation preoperatively and provide postoperative medical management. Optimal care for the surgical patient is realized with a team approach that coordinates the expertise of the hospitalist and the surgical team. Hospitalists apply practice guidelines to medical consultation and can lead initiatives to improve the quality of care and patient safety in the perioperative period.

KNOWLEDGE

Hospitalists should be able to:
- Explain the effect of anesthesia and surgical intervention on physiology.
- Explain the goals and components of preoperative risk assessment.
- Identify patients who require selective preoperative testing based on patient specific factors, type of surgery, and urgency of surgical procedure.
- Describe risk factors for perioperative complications.
- Explain risks for perioperative complications in specific patient populations.
- Explain pharmacologic therapies that should be modified or held prior to surgery.
- List widely accepted risk assessment tools and explain their value and limitations in patients undergoing nonvascular surgery.
- Describe the evidence supporting prophylactic perioperative β-blockade.

SKILLS

Hospitalists should be able to:
- Elicit a thorough history, review the medical record and inquire about functional capacity in patients undergoing surgery.
- Perform a targeted physical examination, focused on the cardiovascular and pulmonary systems and other systems based on patient history.
- Perform a directed and cost effective diagnostic evaluation based on patient relevant history and physical examination findings.
- Employ published algorithms and validated clinical scoring systems, when available, to assess and risk stratify patients.
- Assess the urgency of the requested evaluation and provide feedback and evaluation in an appropriate timeframe.
- Recognize medical conditions that increase risk for perioperative complications and make specific evidence based recommendations to optimize outcomes in the perioperative period.
- Determine the perioperative medical management strategies required to address specific disease states.
- Reassess patients for postoperative complications and make medical recommendations as indicated.

ATTITUDES

Hospitalists should be able to:
- Communicate with patients and families to explain the hospitalist's role in their perioperative medical care, any indicated preoperative testing related to their medical conditions or risk assessment, and any adjustment of pharmacologic therapies.
- Communicate with patients and families to explain any indicated perioperative prophylactic measures.
- Communicate with patients and families to explain the need for follow-up medical care post-discharge.
- Initiate indicated perioperative preventive strategies.
- Recommend specific prophylactic measures, which may include β-blockade, VTE prophylaxis, or aspiration precautions, to avoid complications in the perioperative period.
- Serve as an advocate for patients.
- Promote a collaborative relationship with surgical services, which includes effective communication.

- Assess pain in perioperative patients and make recommendations for pain management when indicated.
- Facilitate discharge planning early in the hospitalization, including communicating with the primary care provider, and presenting the patient and family with contact information for follow-up care.
- Utilize evidence based recommendations for the evaluation and treatment of patients in the perioperative period.

SYSTEM ORGANIZATION AND IMPROVEMENT

To improve efficiency and quality within their organizations, Hospitalists should:
- Lead, coordinate or participate in multidisciplinary efforts to develop clinical guidelines, protocols and pathways to improve the timing and quality of perioperative care from initial preoperative evaluation through all care transitions.
- Lead, coordinate or participate in efforts to improve the efficiency and quality of care through innovative models, which may include co-management of surgical patients in the perioperative period.
- Lead, coordinate or participate in multidisciplinary initiatives to promote patient safety and optimize diagnostic and management strategies for surgical patients requiring medical evaluation.
- Lead, coordinate or participate in multidisciplinary protocols to promote the rapid identification, triage, and expeditious evaluation of patients requiring urgent operations.

SEPSIS SYNDROME

Sepsis syndrome is defined as infection associated with the Systemic Inflammatory Response Syndrome (SIRS). Sepsis has various etiologies and clinical presentations. It accounts for substantial morbidity and mortality. The Healthcare Cost and Utilization Project (HCUP) estimated 300,000 discharges for sepsis syndrome in 2002, with an in-hospital mortality of 18.6%. The mean length-of-stay was 7.3 days with approximately $26,000 in charges per patient. Sepsis requires expeditious diagnosis and standardized treatment plans to favorably impact patient morbidity and mortality. Hospitalists play a key role in the early identification of patients with sepsis, and practice aggressive evidence based evaluation and interventions. Hospitalists lead their institutions to implement early diagnostic strategies, initiate evidence based medical therapies, and incorporate multidisciplinary approaches to the care of patients with sepsis.

KNOWLEDGE

Hospitalists should be able to:
- Define and differentiate bacteremia and the clinical spectrum of SIRS, sepsis, severe sepsis, and septic shock.
- Describe the symptoms and signs of SIRS, sepsis, severe sepsis, and septic shock.
- Describe the inflammatory cascade that leads to SIRS and sepsis.
- Distinguish infectious causes of SIRS from other etiologies.
- Distinguish septic shock from other causes of shock.
- Describe the indicated tests required to evaluate sepsis.
- Identify patient groups with increased risk for the development of sepsis, increased morbidity or mortality, or uncommon etiologic organisms.
- Discuss the evidence based diagnostic choices available in the evaluation of sepsis.
- Describe the indications, contraindications and side effects of therapeutic agents including fluids, vasopressors, antibiotics, steroids, activated protein C, and blood products in the treatment of sepsis.
- Explain indications, contraindications and mechanisms of action of pharmacologic agents used to treat sepsis syndrome.
- Describe the indications for and limitations of central venous access and its value for hemodynamic monitoring and administration of vasoactive agents.
- Describe the role of established scoring systems to estimate the severity of sepsis.
- Explain patient characteristics that on admission portend poor prognosis.
- Explain goals for hospital discharge, including specific measures of clinical stability for safe care transition.

SKILLS

Hospitalists should be able to:
- Utilize all available information, including medical records and history provided by patient and care givers, to identify factors that contribute to the development of sepsis.
- Perform a rapid and targeted physical examination to identify potential sources of sepsis.
- Recognize the value and limitations of the history and physical examination in determining the cause of sepsis.
- Order indicated diagnostic testing to identify the source of sepsis and determine severity of organ dysfunction.
- Rapidly identify patients with septic shock and aggressively treat in parallel with transfer to a critical care setting.
- Assess cardiopulmonary stability and implement aggressive fluid resuscitation, airway maintenance and circulatory support.
- Initiate empiric antimicrobial therapy based on the suspected etiologic source of infection.
- Assess the need for central venous access and monitoring; when needed, coordinate or establish central venous access.
- Determine or coordinate appropriate nutritional and metabolic interventions.
- Support organ function and correct metabolic derangements when indicated.
- Implement measures to ensure strict glycemic control.
- Adopt measures to prevent complications, which may include aspiration precautions, stress ulcer and VTE prophylaxis, and decubitus ulcer prevention.
- Measure and interpret indicated hemodynamic monitoring parameters.

ATTITUDES

Hospitalists should be able to:
- Communicate with patients and families to explain the history and prognosis of sepsis and indicators of functional improvement or decline.
- Communicate with patients and families to explain goals of care plan, including clinical stability criteria, discharge instructions and management after release from hospital.
- Communicate with patients and families to explain tests and procedures and their indications, and to obtain informed consent.
- Recognize the indications for specialty consultations, which may include critical care medicine.
- Employ an early and multidisciplinary approach, which may include respiratory therapy, nursing, pharmacy, nutrition, rehabilitation and social services, that begins at admission and continues through all care transitions.
- Establish and maintain an open dialogue with patients and families regarding care goals and limitations, including palliative care and end-of-life wishes.
- Address resuscitation status early during hospital stay, and discuss and implement end of life decisions by patient or family when indicated or desired.
- Ensure good communication with patients and receiving physicians during care transitions.
- Utilize evidence based recommendations to guide diagnosis, monitoring and treatment of sepsis.

SYSTEM ORGANIZATION AND IMPROVEMENT

To improve efficiency and quality within their organizations, Hospitalists should:
- Lead, coordinate or participate in the development and promotion of guidelines and/or pathways that facilitate efficient and timely evaluation and treatment of patients with sepsis.
- Implement systems to ensure hospital-wide adherence to national standards, and document those measures as specified by recognized organizations.
- Lead, coordinate or participate in multidisciplinary initiatives to promote patient safety and optimize resource utilization.
- Lead, coordinate or participate in intra- and inter-institutional efforts to develop protocols for the rapid identification and transfer of patients with sepsis to appropriate facilities.
- Lead, coordinate or participate in multidisciplinary teams, which may include nutrition, pharmacy, rehabilitation, social services and respiratory therapy, early in the hospital course to improve patient function and outcomes.
- Integrate outcomes research, institution-specific laboratory policies, and hospital formulary to create indicated and cost-effective diagnostic and management strategies for patients with sepsis.

STROKE

Stroke is defined as damage to brain tissue resulting from interruption in blood flow. The American Heart Association (AHA) reports 942,000 discharges for stroke in 2002. Stroke accounted for 1 in 15 deaths in the United States that same year. The average length of stay has been markedly decreasing, but is still almost six days. The estimated direct and indirect cost of stroke in 2005 is $56.8 billion. Stroke care is a rapidly evolving field in which expeditious and careful inpatient care significantly affects outcome. The hospitalist is frequently the primary provider of care for these inpatients. Therefore, it is incumbent on hospitalists to develop the knowledge and skills to identify and manage all types of strokes, coordinate specialty and primary care resources, and guide patients safely and cost-effectively through the acute hospitalization and back into the outpatient setting.

KNOWLEDGE

Hospitalists should be able to:
- Describe the ischemic and hemorrhagic causes of stroke.
- Describe the relationship between the anatomic location of stroke and clinical presentation.
- Employ appropriate imaging and laboratory evaluation to exclude conditions that mimic stroke, guide therapy, and help determine etiology in patients with and without traditional risk factors.
- List risk factors for ischemic and hemorrhagic stroke.
- State indications and contraindications for thrombolytic therapy in the setting of acute stroke.
- Explain indications, contraindications and mechanisms of action of pharmacologic agents used to treat stroke.
- Explain the optimal blood pressure control for individual patients presenting with different types of stroke.
- State indications for early surgical and endovascular interventions.
- Explain the spectrum of functional outcomes of different types of stroke and how these relate to the initial presentation.
- Explain goals for hospital discharge, including specific measures of clinical stability for safe care transition.

SKILLS

Hospitalists should be able to:
- Elicit pertinent details of clinical history and symptoms that are typical of stroke.
- Perform a directed physical examination with emphasis on thorough neurological examination to help guide further evaluation and treatment.
- Diagnose the etiology of stroke through interpretation of initial testing including history, physical examination, electrocardiogram, neurological imaging, and laboratory results.
- Initiate indicated acute therapies to improve the prognosis of stroke.
- Identify patients at risk for acute decompensation, which may include those with signs of increased intracranial pressure and posterior circulation disease, and initiate appropriate therapy.
- Identify patients at risk for aspiration and address nutritional issues.
- Manage the airway when indicated.
- Maintain temperature, blood pressure and glycemic control.
- Assess patients with stroke in a timely manner, and manage or co-manage the patient with the primary requesting service.

ATTITUDES

Hospitalists should be able to:
- Communicate with patients and families to explain the history and prognosis of stroke.
- Communicate with patients and families to explain goals of care plan, discharge instructions and management after release from hospital.
- Communicate with patients and families to explain tests and procedures, and the use and potential side effects of pharmacologic agents.
- Communicate with patients and families to explain the tests and procedures and their indications, and to obtain informed consent.

- Recognize the indications for early specialty consultation, which may include neurology, neurosurgery and interventional radiology.
- Employ prophylaxis against common complications, which may include urinary tract infection, aspiration pneumonia, and venous thromboembolism.
- Initiate secondary stroke prevention.
- Employ an early and multidisciplinary approach to the care of stroke patients that begins at admission and continues through all care transitions.
- Address resuscitation status early during hospital stay; implement end-of-life decisions by patients and/or families when indicated or desired.
- Recognize barriers to follow-up care of stroke patients and involve multidisciplinary hospital staff to accordingly tailor medications and transition of care plans.
- Communicate to outpatient providers the notable events of the hospitalization and post-discharge needs, which may include outpatient cardiac rehabilitation.
- Utilize evidence based recommendations and protocols and risk stratification tools for the treatment of stroke.

SYSTEM ORGANIZATION AND IMPROVEMENT

To improve efficiency and quality within their organizations, Hospitalists should:
- Lead, coordinate or participate in multidisciplinary teams, which may include neurology, rehabilitation medicine, nursing, physical and occupational therapy, speech pathology and other allied health professionals, early in the hospital course to reduce complications, facilitate patient education and discharge planning.
- Lead, coordinate or participate in multidisciplinary efforts to develop protocols to rapidly identify stroke patients with indications for acute interventions and minimize time to intervention.
- Lead, coordinate or participate in multidisciplinary initiatives to promote patient safety and optimize resource utilization, including aggressive treatment of risk factors and rehabilitation.

URINARY TRACT INFECTION

Urinary tract infection (UTI) refers to a spectrum of clinical presentations ranging from asymptomatic urinary infection to acute pyelonephritis with septicemia. UTI is a common infection diagnosed at the time of admission or acquired during hospitalization. According to the Healthcare Cost and Utilization Project (HCUP), the Diagnosis Related Group for UTI with complications or co-morbidities accounted for almost 302,000 hospital discharges in 2002. The mean length-of-stay was 4.9 days with mean charges of $13,000 per patient. In-hospital mortality was 2.2% for this group. Hospitalists diagnose, treat and identify complications of UTI. Hospitalists can lead hospital-wide patient safety initiatives to reduce the incidence of hospital-acquired infection and emerging antibiotic resistance.

KNOWLEDGE

Hospitalists should be able to:
- Define UTI and describe the pathophysiology that leads to complicated UTI.
- Describe common symptoms and signs of UTI.
- Explain the clinical spectrum of UTI including patient populations that may present with atypical symptoms.
- Name common community-acquired and hospital-acquired urinary pathogens.
- Explain how local and national resistance patterns impact the selection of initial antibiotics.
- Distinguish UTI from sterile pyuria and from colonization.
- Explain the indications and limitations of specific tests used to diagnose UTI, its underlying causes and complicating conditions.
- Define risk factors for UTI.
- Name specific patient populations at increased risk for development of hospital acquired or other complicated UTIs.
- Distinguish the specific clinical management, including antibiotic selection for different patient populations, including patients with community-acquired UTI, hospital-acquired UTI, chronic indwelling catheters, pregnancy, immunosuppression and incidentally recognized UTI.
- Explain the indications for hospitalization.
- Explain goals for hospital discharge, including specific measures of clinical stability for safe care transition.

SKILLS

Hospitalists should be able to:
- Elicit a targeted history to identify risk factors and symptoms for UTI and its known complications.
- Perform a focused physical examination looking for signs of complicated UTI, prostatitis and other co-morbid conditions.
- Order and interpret urinalysis and urine culture.
- Order and interpret the results of imaging studies when indicated.
- Formulate an initial care plan based on patient risk factors, acute medical illness, co-morbid disease, and local and national antibiotic resistance patterns.
- Adjust antibiotic therapy based on subsequent culture results and determine appropriate duration of treatment.
- Recognize and address complications of UTI and/or inadequate response to therapy.
- Evaluate and treat patients for UTI in the perioperative setting when indicated.

ATTITUDES

Hospitalists should be able to:
- Communicate with patients and families to explain the goals of care plan, discharge instructions and management after release from hospital.
- Communicate with patients and families to explain tests and procedures, and the use and potential side effects of pharmacologic agents.
- Recognize indications for specialty consultation, which may include urology or infectious disease services.
- Promote and employ prevention measures, which may include early removal of urinary catheters and other interventions to prevent recurrent UTI.

- Apply judicious antibiotic selection to help reduce antibiotic resistance.
- Employ a multidisciplinary approach to the care of patients with complicated UTI that begins on admission and continues through all care transitions.
- Appreciate and treat patient's pain.
- Document treatment plan, and provide clear discharge instructions for the receiving primary care physician, including duration of antibiotic treatment and need for follow-up testing.
- Provide and coordinate resources to patients to ensure safe transition from the hospital to arranged follow-up care.
- Coordinate discharge plans when patients will require ongoing skilled nursing care.
- Utilize evidence based recommendations for the diagnosis and treatment of UTI.

SYSTEM ORGANIZATION AND IMPROVEMENT

To improve efficiency and quality within their organizations, Hospitalists should:
- Implement systems to ensure hospital-wide adherence to national standards, and document those measures as specified by recognized organizations.
- Collaborate with local infection control practitioners to reduce the spread of resistant organisms within the institution.
- Lead, coordinate or participate in multidisciplinary initiatives to minimize use and duration of urinary catheters and reduce incidence of hospital-acquired UTI.

VENOUS THROMBOEMBOLISM

Venous thromboembolism (VTE), or clotting within the venous system, is a common and under-recognized cause of significant preventable morbidity and mortality in hospitalized patients. VTE includes deep vein thrombosis (DVT) and pulmonary embolus (PE). The American Heart Association states that first VTE occurs in roughly 100 patients per 100,000 each year. Of these, one-third have pulmonary embolism. Thirty percent of the 200,000 new cases of VTE annually die within three days, and one-fifth die suddenly due to pulmonary embolus. DVT accounts for approximately 8,000 hospital discharges per year, while PE accounts for almost 100,000 discharges. Hospitalists can lead their institutions in the development of screening and prevention protocols for patients at risk for VTE, and in the promotion of early diagnosis and safe approaches to the treatment of VTE. Hospitalists can also develop strategies to operationalize cost-effective programs that will improve patient outcomes and reduce the economic burden of VTE.

KNOWLEDGE

Hospitalists should be able to:
- Describe VTE pathophysiology, including contributing aspects of endothelial damage, stasis, and alteration of the coagulation cascade.
- Describe the epidemiology of VTE, including the effects of demographic, environmental, thrombophilic, and hormonal factors; underlying medical and surgical conditions, and length of stay.
- Explain the clinical presentation of VTE and describe the diagnostic algorithmic approach.
- Describe the indications and limitations of specific diagnostic tests, including plasma D-Dimer testing, Doppler ultrasound, PE-protocol chest CT, CT of the pelvis and lower extremities, V/Q scanning, and MRI.
- Explain when invasive testing, including pulmonary angiography and venography, is indicated and describe the contraindications and potential complications of such testing.
- Describe the role of additional tests in the assessment of disease severity, including echocardiogram, troponin, and BNP.
- Describe VTE prophylaxis regimens for specific hospitalized risk groups, including medical, general surgical, orthopaedic, neurosurgical, obstetric, ICU, and renal insufficiency patients.
- Describe the indications, contraindications and side effects of thrombolytic therapy in the setting of VTE.
- Explain indications, contraindications and mechanisms of action of pharmacologic agents used to treat VTE.
- Explain the role and potential side effects of other therapeutic modalities in the setting of VTE, including different anticoagulation regimens, IVC filters, and embolectomy.
- Describe poor prognostic factors that necessitate early specialty consultation.
- Explain the indications for hospitalization and admission to the intensive care unit.
- Explain goals for hospital discharge, including specific measures of clinical stability for safe care transition.

SKILLS

Hospitalists should be able to:
- Elicit a thorough and relevant history and review the medical record to identify relevant risk factors and symptoms consistent with VTE.
- Perform a complete physical examination to identify clinical features that predict the presence of VTE and significant clot burden, including evidence of pulmonary hypertension, right heart failure, low perfusion state and underlying malignancy.
- Analyze history and physical findings to determine pretest probability for DVT and/or PE.
- Apply pretest probability and interpretation of diagnostic testing to establish the diagnosis or exclusion of VTE or need for additional testing strategies.
- Determine appropriate level of inpatient care required.
- Appraise the need for urgent invasive treatment modalities, including catheter-directed thrombolysis of the venous or pulmonary artery system, or catheter-directed or surgical embolectomy.

- Formulate a treatment plan tailored to the individual patient, including selection of a specific anticoagulation regimen (agent, dosing, target level and duration) and required monitoring and/or IVC filter placement.
- Anticipate and address factors that may complicate the VTE or its management including cardiopulmonary compromise, bleeding and/or anticoagulation failure.
- Facilitate co-management of VTE treatment and prophylaxis when requested by other services.

ATTITUDES

Hospitalists should be able to:
- Communicate with patients and families to explain the natural history and prognosis of VTE.
- Communicate with patients and families to explain goals of care plan, discharge instructions and management after release from hospital.
- Communicate with patients and families to explain tests and procedures, and the use and potential side effects of pharmacologic agents.
- Communicate with patients and families to explain tests and procedures and their indications, and to obtain informed consent.
- Recognize the need for early specialty consultation, which may include interventional radiology, vascular surgery, and hematology.
- Perform VTE risk assessment in all hospitalized patients and initiate indicated prophylactic measures including pharmacologic agents, mechanical devices and/or ambulation, to reduce the likelihood of VTE.
- Educate clinicians and nurses in VTE risk assessment and preventive measures.
- Employ a multidisciplinary approach, which may include nursing, anticoagulation, pharmacy and nutrition services, to the care of patients with VTE that begins at admission and continues through all care transitions.
- Address and manage pain in patients with VTE.
- Collaborate with primary care physicians and emergency physicians in making the admission decision.
- Document treatment plan and provide clear discharge instructions for receiving primary care physician responsible for monitoring anticoagulation.
- Insure adequate resources, including monitoring of anticoagulation, for patients between hospital discharge and arranged outpatient follow-up.
- Recognize when to prescribe extended duration prophylaxis to patients being discharged to rehabilitation hospitals, skilled nursing facilities, or home with immobility.
- Utilize evidence based recommendations when managing hospitalized patients at risk for VTE or with acute VTE.

SYSTEM ORGANIZATION AND IMPROVEMENT

To improve efficiency and quality within their organizations, Hospitalists should:
- Lead, coordinate or participate in multidisciplinary initiatives to implement screening and prevention protocols for hospitalized patients based on national evidence based recommendations.
- Lead, coordinate or participate in multidisciplinary teams to develop early treatment protocols.
- Lead, coordinate or participate in multidisciplinary initiatives to improve inpatient care efficiency, facilitate early discharge, and encourage the outpatient management of VTE.
- Advocate for the establishment and support of resources to facilitate early discharge including patient education, adequate availability of pharmacologic agents, and home health resources.
- Integrate outcomes research, institution-specific laboratory policies, and hospital formulary to create indicated and cost-effective diagnostic and management strategies for patients with VTE.

Section 2:   PROCEDURES

2.1   Arthrocentesis
2.2   Chest Radiograph Interpretation
2.3   Electrocardiogram Interpretation
2.4   Emergency Procedures
2.5   Lumbar Puncture
2.6   Paracentesis
2.7   Thoracentesis
2.8   Vascular Access

ARTHROCENTESIS

Arthrocentesis, the aspiration of synovial fluid from a joint, is frequently performed in the diagnosis and management of joint effusions. These effusions are associated with infectious, traumatic, and rheumatologic conditions. The Healthcare Cost and Utilization Project (HCUP) reports that arthrocentesis was performed in 32,961 hospitalized patients in 2002. Hospitalists may identify a joint effusion during the history and physical examination, and should use clinical expertise and evidence based decision making to determine whether arthrocentesis is required in the diagnosis and management of the patient's illness.

KNOWLEDGE

Hospitalists should be able to:
- Identify and locate anatomic landmarks to guide proper entry points for arthrocentesis.
- Define and differentiate the disease processes that may lead to the development of joint effusion.
- Explain the indications and contraindications for arthrocentesis, including potential risks and complications.
- Explain the appropriate diagnostic testing for synovial fluid.
- Describe indications for use of ultrasonography to guide arthrocentesis.
- Select the necessary equipment to perform an arthrocentesis at the bedside.

SKILLS

Hospitalists should be able to:
- Distinguish between the clinical features of a joint effusion and soft tissue swelling surrounding a joint.
- Demonstrate the optimal position for the patient and the patient's joint during an arthrocentesis.
- Select and use the correct equipment for a given joint.
- Use sterile techniques during preparation for and performance of arthrocentesis.
- Maintain clinician safety with appropriate protective wear.
- Manage the complications of arthrocentesis.
- Order radiographic studies and interpret findings.
- Order and interpret results of synovial fluid cell count, differential, crystal morphology, gram stain and culture.
- Order and interpret platelet and coagulation studies when indicated.
- Develop management plan based on results of fluid testing.

ATTITUDES

Hospitalists should be able to:
- Communicate with patients and families to explain the procedure, its expected diagnostic or therapeutic benefits, recovery period, and potential and expected outcomes; and to obtain informed consent.
- Discuss with patients and families pain management strategies for discomfort during and after arthrocentesis.
- Relieve pain with splinting and analgesia targeted to the joint inflammation.
- Employ multidisciplinary teams, including physical and occupational therapy when appropriate, to assist with inpatient and outpatient rehabilitation.
- Recognize indications for specialty consultation, which may include rheumatology, orthopaedics or infectious disease.
- Consider early consultation in the management of effusion in a prosthetic joint.

SYSTEM ORGANIZATION AND IMPROVEMENT

To improve efficiency and quality within their organizations, Hospitalists should:

- Lead, coordinate or participate in multidisciplinary initiatives to promote patient safety and optimize resource utilization.
- Lead, coordinate or participate in efforts to develop strategies to minimize institutional complication rates.
- Lead, coordinate or participate in quality improvement programs to monitor hospitalists' performance and/or supervision of arthrocentesis.
- Lead, coordinate or participate in efforts to organize and consolidate arthrocentesis equipment in an identifiable location in the hospital, easily assessable to clinicians who perform the procedure.

CHEST RADIOGRAPH INTERPRETATION

Chest radiographs (CXRs) utilize low-level radiation to form images of the chest anatomy. They are non-invasive and readily available. CXRs are an integral part of the initial evaluation of cardiopulmonary pathology. Hospitalists interpret the results of CXRs, often before radiologists, to diagnose disease and develop treatment plans in hospitalized patients.

KNOWLEDGE

Hospitalists should be able to:
- Explain the normal anatomy of the thorax with particular attention to spatial relationships.
- Explain the images seen on a CXR, including bone and soft tissue structures, airway, lungs, cardiac structure and silhouette, aorta, and diaphragm.
- List the indications for ordering a CXR.
- Describe evidence based national guidelines for ordering CXRs.
- Compare the diagnostic utility and limitations of portable radiographs to posteroanterior and lateral radiographs.
- Explain the indications for a lateral decubitus CXR.
- Describe the effects of film exposure, inspiratory effort, and patient position on the radiographic image.
- Explain the effect of cardiovascular, systemic, and traumatic processes on the CXR.
- Explain the limitations of various CXR findings.

SKILLS

Hospitalists should be able to:
- Review a CXR utilizing a systemic approach.
- Identify normal variants.
- Identify abnormalities shown on a CSR and, when possible, correlate with clinical presentation and/or prior procedures.
- Correlate physical examination findings with CXR abnormalities.
- Synthesize CXR findings with other clinical and diagnostic information to diagnose disease and develop a clinical plan.

ATTITUDES

Hospitalists should be able to:
- Communicate with patients and families to explain results of CXRs and how the findings influence the care plan.
- Personally and promptly interpret CXRs and compare them to previously obtained CXRs, when available.
- Review each CXR with a standard and consistent approach.
- Consult and collaborate with radiologists in interpreting complex CXRs and in ordering further diagnostic studies or procedures based on CXR interpretation.
- Utilize evidence based national guidelines to ensure cost efficiency and to minimize unnecessary patient imaging.

SYSTEM ORGANIZATION AND IMPROVEMENT

To improve quality and efficiency within their organizations, Hospitalists should:
- Lead, coordinate or participate in efforts to develop protocols to minimize unnecessary CXRs.
- Identify and convey the need for system improvements related to acquisition and interpretation of CXRs for hospitalized patients.

ELECTROCARDIOGRAM INTERPRETATION

Heart disease continues to be the leading cause of hospital admissions and mortality in the United States, accounting for an estimated 13% of admissions in 2001, and 21% of in-hospital deaths in 2000. The electrocardiogram (EKG), a graphical representation of cardiac electrical potentials, is a noninvasive, readily available diagnostic tool. It remains the most commonly used investigative modality for the initial evaluation of cardiovascular disease. Hospitalists interpret these results expediently and apply the results to estimate risk, diagnose disease, and determine therapeutic needs in the hospitalized patient.

KNOWLEDGE

Hospitalists should be able to:
- Explain the anatomy and physiology of normal and pathologic cardiac tissues, including spatial relationships, vascular supply, automaticity, conduction, and autonomic innervations and how these affect EKG interpretation.
- Compare the diagnostic utility of rhythm strips and telemetry monitors to 12-lead EKG.
- Explain indications for ordering an EKG, including right-sided EKG.
- Describe the implications of the acquisition, amplification, display, and standardization of electrocardiographic waveforms in different leads.
- Describe the relevant components of the EKG tracing.
- Explain the effect of cardiovascular, metabolic, toxic, and systemic disease processes on cardiac electrical potentials of the EKG.
- Explain the limitations of various EKG findings, including computerized interpretations.

SKILLS

Hospitalists should be able to:
- Demonstrate correct lead placement.
- Accurately measure and interpret the atrial and ventricular rates, voltages and intervals of EKG tracings.
- Recognize normal EKG findings, including variations associated with demographics, artifact, lead placement, and other technical problems.
- Recognize and categorize abnormal EKG findings, including abnormalities of conduction, automaticity, anatomy, and manifestations of non-cardiac disease.
- Identify paced rhythms and describe the limitations of related EKG interpretations.
- Synthesize EKG data with other clinical information to risk stratify patients and develop a clinical plan.

ATTITUDES

Hospitalists should be able to:
- Communicate with patients and families to explain results of the EKG and how the findings impact the care plan.
- Personally and promptly interpret EKGs and compare them to previously recorded EKGs, when available.
- Review each EKG with a standard and consistent approach.
- Consult and collaborate with cardiologists in interpreting complex EKGs, and in ordering further diagnostic studies or procedures based on EKG interpretation.
- Determine the need for specialist intervention based on the urgency and patient risk.

SYSTEM ORGANIZATION AND IMPROVEMENT

To improve quality and efficiency within their organizations, Hospitalists should:
- Lead, coordinate or participate in efforts to expedite acquisition and interpretation of EKGs for hospitalized patients.

EMERGENCY PROCEDURES

In Hospital Medicine, emergency procedures refer to advanced cardiac life support (ACLS), endotracheal intubation, and short-term mechanical ventilation. Hospitalists care for patients admitted to the hospital with critical illnesses, as well as patients who have become critically ill during their hospital stay. In providing care to patients who have become critically ill, many Hospitalists perform or supervise these emergency procedures. Hospitalists lead efforts to provide timely, standardized response to inpatient emergencies.

CARDIOPULMONARY RESUSCITATION

KNOWLEDGE

Hospitalists should be able to:
- Describe the normal anatomy of the oral cavity, airway, thorax, heart and lungs.
- Describe the clinical findings or disease processes that require implementation of cardiopulmonary resuscitation and advanced life support.
- Describe clinical or cardiac rhythm findings that may impact outcomes for patients with cardiopulmonary arrest.
- List the laboratory and other diagnostic tests indicated during cardiopulmonary distress or arrest and immediately following successful resuscitation.
- Explain basic life support (BLS) protocols.
- Explain and differentiate current ACLS protocols, including the indicated interventions, based on the clinical situation and cardiac rhythm.
- Select the necessary equipment to manage the airway, identify cardiac rhythms, and perform defibrillation.
- Explain which cardiac rhythms and clinical situations require immediate defibrillation.
- Explain the mechanisms of action and uses of medications employed during ACLS.
- Explain the indications for procedural interventions that may be employed during the course of resuscitation.
- Explain the role of hyperthermia as a neuro-protective measure in the post-resuscitation period.

SKILLS

Hospitalists should be able to:
- Promptly identify acute cardiopulmonary distress or arrest, and call for assistance.
- Assess the patient, rapidly review the situation, and develop a differential diagnosis of etiology.
- Elicit additional history from the patient's family, other healthcare providers, and the patient's chart when available.
- Clearly and rapidly identify the event leader, and delineate other staff roles at the beginning of the resuscitation event.
- Properly position the patient on a backboard to perform BLS and ACLS protocols.
- Continually reassess proper patient positioning during resuscitation.
- Perform BLS protocols to open the airway, use a bag-valve-mask ventilatory device, and perform external chest compressions.
- Attach a defibrillator/pacer pads to the patient, and explain the operation of manual and automated defibrillators and external pacing systems.
- Maintain clinician safety with appropriate protective wear.
- Interpret cardiac rhythms and other diagnostic indicators.
- Synthesize diagnostic information to deliver medications and/or defibrillation, and perform procedures required during resuscitation efforts.

ATTITUDES

Hospitalists should be able to:
- Assess and respect the wishes of patients and families who desire no or limited resuscitation measures during hospitalization.
- Communicate with families to explain the efforts performed as well as outcomes and next steps.
- Rapidly respond to emergencies without distraction.

- Facilitate interactions between healthcare professionals about the roles that each will perform during the resuscitation effort.
- Review the resuscitation documentation for accuracy immediately following the event.
- Recognize the indications for emergent specialty consultation when available, which may include ENT, surgery, or critical care medicine.
- Appreciate the value of spiritual support services during and following resuscitation efforts.
- Discontinue resuscitation efforts when interventions have been unsuccessful and continued efforts are medically futile.
- Arrange for appropriate care transitions following successful resuscitation.
- Address family wishes regarding organ donation and autopsy.

ENDOTRACHEAL INTUBATION

KNOWLEDGE

Hospitalists should be able to:
- Describe the anatomy of the oral cavity, posterior pharynx and larynx.
- Describe clinical findings or disease processes that may require securing an airway.
- Describe the indications and contraindications, benefits and risks of endotracheal intubation.
- Describe the necessary equipment and medications required for routine and difficult intubations.
- Describe the process of endotracheal intubation from laryngoscope assembly to assessment of tube placement.
- Describe and differentiate alternatives to endotracheal intubation.

SKILLS

Hospitalists should be able to:
- Identify patients for whom endotracheal intubation may be required.
- Utilize bag-valve-mask ventilation with oral or nasal airway as a bridge to intubation.
- Select the appropriate laryngoscope blade for the individual patient.
- Position the patient and the bed for optimal procedure success and operator comfort.
- Assemble the laryngoscope and intubate the patient after visualizing the vocal cords.
- Prepare the oropharynx for intubation using necessary steps that may include removal of oral hardware, suctioning, and application of cricoid pressure.
- Request cricoid pressure and other maneuvers when indicated.
- Place the endotracheal tube at an appropriate depth in the airway.
- Confirm endotracheal tube placement by gastric and breath sounds, carbon dioxide monitor, and radiography; adjust tube position when indicated.

ATTITUDES

Hospitalists should be able to:
- Communicate with patients and families regarding procedure indications and next steps in management.
- Maintain high oxygen saturation prior to intubation whenever possible.
- Minimize patient trauma risk during intubations.
- Appreciate that bag-valve-mask can provide adequate oxygenation for extended periods when difficult intubations are delayed.
- Maintain clinician safety with appropriate protective wear.
- Use an alternative airway control device (e.g. laryngeal mask airway) for patients with difficult or unsuccessful intubations.
- Request appropriate specialist consultation for difficult or unsuccessful intubations or when clinician experience level precludes intubation trial.

MECHANICAL VENTILATION

KNOWLEDGE

Hospitalists should be able to:
- Describe the normal anatomy of the chest wall, thorax, and lung.
- Describe disease processes that lead to respiratory failure and expected clinical findings.
- Describe the indications, benefits and risks of mechanical ventilation.
- Describe indications and contraindications for non-invasive ventilation in selected patients.
- Explain the role of arterial blood gas (ABG) analysis in the management of ventilated patients.
- Describe available modes of ventilation, and how to select initial and subsequent ventilator settings.
- Describe methods of and indications for sedation, comfort management, and/or paralysis in ventilated patients.
- Describe various ventilator settings and explain the use of individual settings based on the patient's disease process and clinical condition.

SKILLS

Hospitalists should be able to:
- Utilize nursing and respiratory therapy reports, physical examination, and ventilator data to identify complications due to mechanical ventilation.
- Select and adjust the ventilator mode and settings based on underlying disease process, other patient factors, ventilator data, and ABG analysis.
- Employ indicated interventions when complications of mechanical ventilation are identified.
- Identify the components of the ventilator, assess proper functioning, and identify equipment malfunction and/or patient-ventilator dysynchrony.
- Order and interpret laboratory and imaging studies based on changes in patient's clinical status.
- Order adequate sedation and other indicated interventions to treat underlying conditions leading to respiratory failure and to prevent the complications of mechanical ventilation.

ATTITUDES

Hospitalists should be able to:
- Communicate with patients and/or families to explain the risks, benefits, and alternatives to invasive ventilation.
- Obtain informed consent prior to non-emergent intubations.
- Conduct regular family meetings to provide clinical updates and facilitate shared decision-making.
- Implement interventions shown to reduce risk of ventilator-associated complications, which may include hospital acquired pneumonia, stress ulceration and bleeding, and venous thromboembolism.
- Provide adequate sedation, comfort management, and paralysis when indicated for patients requiring mechanical ventilation.
- Recognize the indications for specialty consultation, which may include critical care medicine.

SYSTEM ORGANIZATION AND IMPROVEMENT FOR EMERGENCY PROCEDURES

To improve efficiency and quality within their organizations, Hospitalists should:
- Collaborate with critical care physicians, respiratory therapists, and critical care nurses to develop evidence based protocols or guidelines for optimal ventilator management and weaning.
- Lead, coordinate or participate in evaluation of resuscitation and mechanical ventilation outcomes and identify and implement improvement initiatives.
- Lead, coordinate or participate in multidisciplinary teams, which may include critical care nurses, respiratory therapists, and critical care and emergency physicians, to establish ongoing training to ensure high quality performance of emergency procedures.
- Lead, coordinate or participate in multidisciplinary efforts to review antecedent events to identify changes in clinical status which, if promptly identified and acted upon, may have prevented the emergency intervention.
- Facilitate appropriate organization and consolidation of equipment in multiple identifiable and accessible locations in the hospital for performance of emergency procedures.

LUMBAR PUNCTURE

Lumbar puncture is a procedure during which a needle is inserted into the subarachnoid space to obtain cerebrospinal fluid (CSF) for laboratory analysis. CSF is formed within the ventricular choroid plexus and distributed in the ventricular system, basal cisterns and the subarachnoid space. The Healthcare Cost and Utilization Project (HCUP) estimates over 240,000 lumbar punctures were performed in hospitalized patients in 2002. Hospitalists identify patients who require lumbar puncture to assess acute or chronic central nervous system (CNS) disease processes. Early diagnosis and therapy of acute CNS infections or subarachnoid hemorrhage is essential to lower morbidity and mortality.

KNOWLEDGE

Hospitalists should be able to:
- Describe the anatomy of the spinal column and the spinal cord.
- Describe the signs and symptoms that require lumbar puncture.
- Describe disease processes that require frequent therapeutic lumbar puncture.
- Explain the indications and contraindications for lumbar puncture, including potential risks and complications.
- Describe the physical examination maneuvers used in the evaluation of suspected CNS infections and identify their sensitivity and specificity.
- List the indications for brain imaging prior to lumbar puncture.
- Explain the diagnostic testing indicated for CSF based on the clinical presentation.
- Describe indications for the use of interventional radiology in performing lumber puncture.
- Select the necessary equipment to perform a lumbar puncture at the bedside.

SKILLS

Hospitalists should be able to:
- Elicit a thorough history and review medical records to identify indications and potential contraindications for lumbar puncture.
- Perform a thorough physical examination, including neurologic and fundoscopic examination.
- Properly position the patient for lumbar puncture and identify major anatomic landmarks.
- Use sterile techniques during preparation for and performance of lumbar puncture.
- Obtain an accurate measurement of and interpret the opening pressure.
- Maintain clinician safety with appropriate protective wear.
- Manage the complications of lumbar puncture, particularly post-lumbar puncture headache.
- Order and interpret indicated diagnostic tests for CSF fluid.
- Order and interpret platelet and coagulation studies when indicated.
- Synthesize data obtained from history, physical examination, radiographic imaging, and CSF analysis to develop an evidence based treatment plan.

ATTITUDES

Hospitalists should be able to:
- Communicate with patients and families to explain the procedure, its expected diagnostic benefits, and potential complications; and to obtain informed consent.
- Discuss with patients and families pain management strategies for discomfort during and after lumbar puncture.
- Recognize the importance of proper positioning following the procedure.
- Identify patients who require isolation precautions.
- Manage patient discomfort or pain during and after the procedure.
- Recognize the indications for specialty consultation, which may include interventional radiology, infectious disease or neurology.

SYSTEM ORGANIZATION AND IMPROVEMENT

To improve efficiency and quality within their organizations, Hospitalists should:

- Collaborate with emergency physicians to develop protocols for rapid identification and evaluation of patients with suspected CNS infections.
- Lead, coordinate or participate in efforts to develop strategies to minimize institution complication rates.
- Lead, coordinate or participate in quality improvement programs to monitor hospitalists' performance and/or supervision of lumbar puncture.
- Lead, coordinate or participate in efforts to organize and consolidate lumbar puncture equipment in an identifiable location in the hospital, easily accessible to clinicians who perform the procedure.

PARACENTESIS

Paracentesis, the aspiration of fluid from the abdominal cavity, is a diagnostic and therapeutic procedure frequently performed in the hospital. Paracentesis was performed in almost 90,000 discharges in 2002, according to the Healthcare Cost and Utilization Project (HCUP). Hospitalists identify patients with suspected ascites on the basis of the clinical presentation, physical examination and/or ultrasonography. Utilizing evidence based decision making, hospitalists determine whether paracentesis is indicated in the diagnosis of disease or palliation of patient symptoms.

KNOWLEDGE

Hospitalists should be able to:
- Describe the normal anatomy of the abdomen and pelvis.
- Define and differentiate pathophysiologic processes that may lead to the development of ascites.
- Describe clinical presentations consistent with spontaneous bacterial peritonitis.
- Explain indications and contraindications for paracentesis, including potential risks and complications.
- Describe the physical examination maneuvers used in the evaluation of ascites and identify their sensitivity and specificity.
- Differentiate the indications for a diagnostic paracentesis versus a large-volume paracentesis.
- Explain the appropriate diagnostic testing for ascitic fluid.
- Describe indications for use of ultrasonography to assess the quantity of ascitic fluid and/or to guide paracentesis.
- Select the necessary equipment to perform a paracentesis at the bedside, and differentiate what is needed for a diagnostic versus a large-volume paracentesis.
- Define the serum-ascites albumin gradient and its role in the evaluation of ascites.
- Identify the indications for administration of albumin in conjunction with paracentesis.
- Identify patients with ascites who may benefit from large-volume paracentesis.

SKILLS

Hospitalists should be able to:
- Elicit a thorough and relevant history to identify co-morbid conditions and risk factors for the development or complications of ascites.
- Perform a thorough physical examination, evaluating for signs associated with chronic liver disease or malignancy.
- Perform an abdominal examination, including specific maneuvers to assess for the presence of ascites.
- Properly position the patient and identify anatomic landmarks to perform a paracentesis.
- Use sterile techniques during preparation for and performance of paracentesis.
- Maintain clinician safety with appropriate protective wear.
- Manage the complications of paracentesis following the procedure, which ma include bleeding, persistent leak of ascitic fluid, and hemodynamic compromise.
- Order and interpret the results of ascitic fluid analysis, including cell count, differential, gram stain and culture, and serum-ascites albumin gradient.
- Order and interpret platelet and coagulation studies when indicated.
- Synthesize a management plan based on history, physical examination, radiographic imaging and the results of fluid testing.

ATTITUDES

Hospitalists should be able to:
- Communicate with patients and families to explain the procedure, its expected diagnostic or therapeutic benefits, and potential complications; and to obtain informed consent.
- Manage patient discomfort or pain during and after the procedure.
- Identify patients who may benefit from transfusion of fresh frozen plasma and/or platelets prior to paracentesis.
- Recognize the indications for specialty consultations, which may include interventional radiology or gastroenterology.

SYSTEM ORGANIZATION AND IMPROVEMENT

To improve efficiency and quality within their institutions, Hospitalists should:

- Lead, coordinate or participate in multidisciplinary initiatives to promote patient safety and optimize resource utilization.
- Lead, coordinate or participate in development of institutional guidelines for the pre-procedure utilization of fresh frozen plasma and platelet transfusions in patients with coagulopathy or thrombocytopenia.
- Lead, coordinate or participate in development of institutional guidelines to identify patients who should receive albumin peri-procedure.
- Collaborate with radiologists to standardize identification of patients who would benefit from ultrasound-guided paracentesis.
- Lead, coordinate or participate in efforts to develop strategies to minimize institutional complication rates.
- Lead, coordinate or participate in quality improvement programs to monitor hospitalists' performance and/or supervision of paracentesis.
- Lead, coordinate, or participate in efforts to organize and consolidate paracentesis equipment in an identifiable location in the hospital, easily accessible to clinicians who perform the procedure.

THORACENTESIS

Thoracentesis is a bedside procedure involving the withdrawal of fluid from the pleural cavity. Pleural effusions are associated with several disease processes in hospitalized patients and may be evaluated using thoracentesis. The Healthcare Cost and Utilization Project (HCUP) estimates almost 189,000 thoracenteses were performed in hospitalized patients in 2002, although this total includes chest tube placement as well. Using the history, physical examination and radiographic findings, hospitalists identify those patients who would benefit from diagnostic or therapeutic thoracentesis.

KNOWLEDGE

Hospitalists should be able to:
- Describe the normal anatomy of the chest wall, thorax and lung.
- Define and differentiate the disease processes that may lead to the development of pleural effusion.
- Define and differentiate transudative and exudative pleural effusions and their causes.
- Explain indications and contraindications of thoracentesis and its potential risks and complications.
- Explain the role of chest imaging in the evaluation of pleural effusion.
- Explain the appropriate diagnostic testing for pleural fluid.
- Describe indications for use of ultrasonography or computed tomography to assess the quantity of pleural fluid and/or guide thoracentesis.
- Select the necessary equipment to perform a thoracentesis at the bedside, and differentiate what is needed for diagnostic versus therapeutic thoracentesis.
- Define the criteria that distinguish transudative and exudative effusions.
- Describe the effects of various disease processes on pleural fluid results.

SKILLS

Hospitalists should be able to:
- Elicit a thorough history, identifying potential disease processes and risk factors for the development of pleural effusions.
- Perform a chest examination, including specific maneuvers to assess for the presence of pleural effusion.
- Properly position the patient and identify anatomic landmarks to perform a thoracentesis.
- Use sterile techniques during preparation for and performance of thoracentesis.
- Maintain clinician safety with appropriate protective wear.
- Recognize and manage complications associated with thoracentesis, especially pneumothorax and re-expansion pulmonary edema.
- Order and interpret the results of pleural fluid analysis.
- Order and interpret platelet and coagulation studies when indicated.
- Determine need for chest tube placement based on thoracentesis results.
- Synthesize a management plan based on history, physical examination, radiographic imaging and results of pleural fluid analysis.
- Identify patients with pleural effusions who may benefit from therapeutic thoracentesis, chest tube placement and/or pleurodesis.

ATTITUDES

Hospitalists should be able to:
- Communicate with patients and families to explain the procedure, its expected diagnostic or therapeutic benefits, and potential complications; and to obtain informed consent.
- Order and promptly review the results of routine post-procedure chest radiographs.
- Manage patient discomfort or pain during and after the procedure.
- Recognize indications for specialty consultations, which may include interventional radiology, pulmonary medicine, infectious disease, or cardiothoracic surgery.

SYSTEM ORGANIZATION AND IMPROVEMENT

To improve efficiency and quality within their institutions, Hospitalists should:

- Lead, coordinate or participate in multidisciplinary initiatives to promote patient safety and optimize resource utilization.
- Lead, coordinate or participate in development of institutional guidelines for the pre-procedure utilization of fresh frozen plasma and platelet transfusions in patients with coagulopathy or thrombocytopenia.
- Lead, coordinate or participate in development of institutional guidelines to identify patients who should receive albumin peri-procedure.
- Collaborate with radiologists to standardize identification of patients who would benefit from ultrasound-guided paracentesis.
- Lead, coordinate or participate in efforts to develop strategies to minimize institutional complication rates.
- Lead, coordinate or participate in quality improvement programs to monitor hospitalists' performance and/or supervision of paracentesis.
- Lead, coordinate, or participate in efforts to organize and consolidate paracentesis equipment in an identifiable location in the hospital, easily accessible to clinicians who perform the procedure.

VASCULAR ACCESS

Vascular access involves inserting a catheter into an appropriate blood vessel in order to measure useful diagnostic parameters, draw blood for diagnostic testing, and/or provide specific therapeutic interventions.

Vascular access procedures were performed in approximately 417,000 discharges in 2002, according to the Healthcare Cost and Utilization Project (HCUP). Many hospitalized patients require vascular access, and hospitalists will differentiate patients who simply need peripheral venous access from those who require more invasive types of arterial or central venous access. Complications of vascular catheters can cause prolonged hospital stays and increase morbidity and mortality. Hospitalists advocate for patients to determine the most appropriate type of vascular access based on the patient's diagnostic and therapeutic requirements and overall clinical condition.

KNOWLEDGE

Hospitalists should be able to:
- Name the various locations for peripheral venous access and describe the normal vasculature and surrounding anatomy of the site chosen for access.
- Name the various locations for arterial or central venous access and describe the normal vasculature and surrounding anatomy of the site chosen for vascular access.
- Describe the collateral flow for arterial access procedures.
- Describe the clinical findings or disease processes that require arterial or central venous access.
- Explain the role of ultrasonography in vascular access placement.
- Explain indications and contraindications of the various arterial or central venous access procedures.
- Describe and differentiate the potential risks and complications of individual vascular access procedures based on the site chosen and other risk factors.
- Select the necessary equipment to perform the indicated vascular access procedure at the bedside.

SKILLS

Hospitalists should be able to:
- Elicit an accurate and thorough history to identify co-morbid conditions and risk factors for complications related to arterial or central venous vascular access placement.
- Identify absolute and relative contraindications to placement of arterial access or central venous access at specific sites.
- Perform a directed physical examination of the site(s) intended for vascular access.
- Perform specific maneuvers to evaluate for collateral flow for arterial access procedures.
- Properly position the patient and identify anatomic landmarks to obtain vascular access.
- Use sterile techniques during preparation for and performance of vascular access procedures.
- Anticipate and manage complications from the vascular access procedure and in-dwelling catheter.
- Identify and manage the complications of vascular access procedures, which may include infection, thrombotic, and mechanical complications.
- Order and interpret platelet and coagulation studies when indicated.

ATTITUDES

Hospitalists should be able to:
- Communicate with patients and families to explain the indications and alternatives to vascular access.
- Communicate with patients and families to explain the procedure, its expected therapeutic benefits and potential complications; and to obtain informed consent.
- Provide education to patients and their families regarding the care of long-term vascular access.
- Recognize the importance of proper positioning during the procedure.
- Remove all central venous catheters and arterial catheters as soon as they are no longer needed.
- Promote the use of peripheral venous access over central venous access whenever possible.
- Manage patient discomfort or pain during and after the procedure.

- Recognize the indications for specialty consultation, which may include interventional radiology, surgery, or critical care medicine.
- Arrange appropriate care for patients being discharged with long-term vascular access.

SYSTEM ORGANIZATION AND IMPROVEMENT

To improve efficiency and quality within their organizations, Hospitalists should:
- Lead, coordinate or participate in multidisciplinary initiatives to promote patient safety and optimize resource utilization.
- Lead, coordinate or participate in development of IV access teams to improve the placement and maintenance of IV catheters.
- Lead, coordinator or participate in quality improvement programs to monitor hospitalists' performance and/or supervision of vascular access.
- Lead, coordinate or participate in implementation of standard nursing protocols for catheter care.
- Lead, coordinate or participate in efforts to organize and consolidate equipment in an identifiable location in the hospital that is easily accessible to clinicians who perform the procedure.

Section 3:   **HEALTHCARE SYSTEMS**

3.1   Care of the Elderly Patient
3.2   Care of Vulnerable Populations
3.3   Communication
3.4   Diagnostic Decision Making
3.5   Drug Safety, Pharmacoeconomics and Pharmacoepidemiology
3.6   Equitable Allocation of Resources
3.7   Evidence Based Medicine
3.8   Hospitalist as Consultant
3.9   Hospitalist as Teacher
3.10   Information Management
3.11   Leadership
3.12   Management Practices
3.13   Nutrition and the Hospitalized Patient
3.14   Palliative Care
3.15   Patient Education
3.16   Patient Handoff
3.17   Patient Safety
3.18   Practice Based Learning and Improvement
3.19   Prevention of Healthcare Associated Infections and Antimicrobial Resistance
3.20   Professionalism and Medical Ethics
3.21   Quality Improvement
3.22   Risk Management
3.23   Team Approach and Multidisciplinary Care
3.24   Transitions of Care

CARE OF THE ELDERLY PATIENT

Patients age 65 years or older represent over 30% of acute care hospitalizations and 50% of hospital expenditures. The hospitalized elder is at risk for a multitude of poor outcomes, which may include increased mortality, prolonged length of stay, high rates of readmission, skilled nursing facility placement, and delirium and functional decline. These outcomes have significant medical, psychosocial, and economic impact on individual patients and families as well as on the healthcare system in general. In addition to disease-based management, care of the elderly must be approached within a specific psychosocial and functional context. Hospitalists engage in a collaborative, multidisciplinary approach to the care of elderly patients that begins at the time of hospital admission and continues through all care transitions. Hospitalists can lead initiatives that improve the care of elderly patients.

KNOWLEDGE

Hospitalists should be able to:
- Describe the complications related to hospitalization in the elderly.
- Describe the environmental or iatrogenic factors that may contribute to complications in the hospitalized elderly.
- List medications with potential to cause adverse drug reactions in the elderly.
- Describe interventions that can decrease rates of poor outcomes in the hospitalized elderly.
- Explain the key elements of the discharge planning process and options for post-acute care.
- Describe the multiple options for transition from the acute care hospital that can assist patients in regaining functional capacity.
- List patient-specific risk factors for complications in the hospitalized elderly.

SKILLS

Hospitalists should be able to:
- Perform a thorough history and physical examination to identify patient risk factors for complications during hospitalization.
- Perform a brief cognitive and functional assessment of the elderly patient.
- Use active measures to prevent, identify, evaluate and treat pressure ulcers.
- Formulate multidisciplinary care plans for the prevention of delirium, falls, and functional decline.
- Provide non-pharmacologic alternatives for the management of agitation, insomnia, and delirium.
- Prescribe medications for the behavioral symptoms of delirium or dementia that cannot be controlled with non-pharmacologic management.
- Perform a social assessment of the patient's living conditions/support systems and understand how that impacts the patient's health and care plan.
- Formulate safe multidisciplinary plans for care transitions for elderly patients with complex discharge needs.
- Incorporate unique characteristics of elderly patients into the development of therapeutic plans.
- Recognize signs of potential elder abuse.

ATTITUDES

Hospitalists should be able to:
- Appreciate the complications and potential adverse effects associated with polypharmacy.
- Educate patients and families about individual measures and community resources that can reduce potential complications after discharge.
- Appreciate the risks and complications associated with restraint use.
- Appreciate the concept of transitional care.
- Participate actively in multidisciplinary team meetings to formulate coordinated care plans for acute hospitalization and care transitions.
- Promote a team approach to the care of the hospitalized elder, which may include physicians, nurses, pharmacists, social workers, and rehabilitation services.
- Appreciate the medical, psychosocial and economic impact of hospitalization on elderly patients and their families.

- Establish and maintain an open dialogue with patients and families regarding care goals and limitations, palliative care, and end of life issues, including living wills.
- Connect elderly patients with social services early in the hospital course to provide institutional support, which may include referral for insurance and drug benefits, transportation, mental health services and substance abuse services.
- Communicate effectively with primary care physicians and other post-acute care providers to promote safe, coordinated care transitions.
- Lead, coordinate or participate in multidisciplinary hospital initiatives to develop prevention programs and standardized treatment algorithms for elder outcomes such as delirium, falls, functional decline, and pressure ulcers.
- Lead, coordinate or participate in hospital initiatives to improve care transitions and reduce poor discharge outcomes in the elderly.
- Lead, coordinate or participate in patient safety initiatives to reduce common elder complications in the hospital.

CARE OF VULNERABLE POPULATIONS

Vulnerable populations are defined as groups who are at increased risk of receiving a disparity in medical care on the basis of financial circumstances or social characteristics such as age, race, gender, ethnicity, sexual orientation, spirituality, disability, or socioeconomic or insurance status. Hospitalists may play a significant role in influencing the health status, health care access, and health care delivery to vulnerable populations due to their higher rates of hospital utilization and lower access to outpatient care. Agency for Healthcare Research and Quality (AHRQ) estimates health expenditures due to low health literacy range from $29 billion to $69 billion per year. Death rates per 1,000 admissions in low mortality Diagnosis Related Groups (DRG) are higher for hispanics (0.65), blacks (0.71) and the uninsured (1.1) compared to whites (0.61) and the privately insured (0.61). The Nationwide Inpatient Sample (NIS) benchmark mortality in low mortality DRGs is less than 0.5%. Hospitalists may serve as initial points of contact for the health care of these groups. Core competencies in communication, advocacy and comprehension of the health care needs of vulnerable populations may influence healthcare expenditures, morbidity and mortality. Hospitalists can lead initiatives that promote equity of healthcare provision.

KNOWLEDGE

Hospitalists should be able to:
- Explain key factors leading to disparities in health status among specific vulnerable populations.
- Explain disease processes that disproportionately affect vulnerable populations.
- Describe key factors leading to disparities in the quality of care provided to vulnerable groups.
- List services in local healthcare system designed to ameliorate barriers to care provision.
- Name local and institutional resources available to patients needing financial assistance.
- Identify key elements of discharge planning for uninsured, underinsured, and disabled patients.

SKILLS

Hospitalists should be able to:
- Elicit elements of the history and physical examination to detect illnesses for which vulnerable populations may have increased risk.
- Elicit a social history to assess patient habits, identify patients at risk for breaks in transitions of care, and clarify patient values around treatment options.
- Tailor the therapeutic plan that takes into account discharge plan and outpatient resources.
- Identify vulnerable patients whose outpatient environment might benefit from additional community resources.
- Target vulnerable groups for indicated vaccinations and preventive care services or referrals.

ATTITUDES

Hospitalists should be able to:
- Utilize appropriate educational resources to inform vulnerable patients with low health literacy.
- Provide education and systems interventions to minimize medication errors in patients with low health literacy.
- Communicate openly to facilitate trust in patient-physician interactions.
- Actively involve patients and families in the design of care plans.
- Secure translators to assist with interviewing, physical examination, and medical decision making.
- Facilitate communication between vulnerable patient groups and consultants.
- Provide leadership to foster attitudes and systems improvements that promote quality health care provision to vulnerable populations.
- Connect vulnerable patients with social services early in the hospital course to provide institutional support, which may include referral for insurance and drug benefits, transportation, mental health services and substance abuse services.
- Coordinate adequate transitions of care from the inpatient to outpatient setting.
- Communicate with primary care physicians to facilitate transitions of care.

COMMUNICATION

Communication refers the transfer of information between individuals, groups, or organizations. Hospitalists communicate in multiple modalities with patients, families, other health care providers and administrators. Patient-centered care requires that physicians and members of multidisciplinary teams effectively inform, educate, reassure, and empower patients and families to participate in the creation of a care plan. Effective communication is central to the role of the hospitalist to promote efficient, safe, and high quality care and to reduce discontinuity of care. Hospitalists can lead initiatives to improve communication amongst team members, patients, families, primary care physicians and receiving physicians within the hospital and at extended care facilities beginning with admission and through all care transitions.

KNOWLEDGE

Hospitalists should be able to:
- Describe key elements in a message.
- Describe various modalities used to communicate, including advantages and disadvantages of each.
- Describe techniques of providing and eliciting feedback, and differentiate formative and summative feedback.
- Define the role of effective communication in risk management.

SKILLS

Hospitalists should be able to:
- Explain issues of pathophysiology, treatment options, and prognosis using language understandable to patients, family members, and other care providers.
- Listen without interruption to the questions and concerns of patients, family members and other care providers, and promptly address any issues.
- Identify potentially problematic family and team dynamics and explore their effects on the patient.
- Identify a family spokesperson.
- Facilitate family meetings when necessary, collaborating with nurses and other team members to identify goals for the meeting, summarize conclusions reached, and utilize support staff as needed.
- Effectively utilize a translator when communicating with patients and families speaking a different language.

ATTITUDES

Hospitalists should be able to:
- Appreciate the positive impact that subtle changes in body language, such as sitting and appropriate touching, have on patient and family perceptions of an interaction.
- Demonstrate empathy for patient and family concerns.
- Recognize the importance of allowing patients and families to have questions answered in a straightforward and timely manner.
- Demonstrate cultural sensitivity in all interactions with patients and families.
- Appreciate the importance of active listening.
- Counsel patients and families objectively when considering various treatment options.
- Acknowledge and remain comfortable with uncertainty in issues of prognosis.
- Provide a quiet and comfortable setting for family meetings.
- Discuss the patient's illness realistically without negating hope.
- Ensure that input from surrogate decision makers accurately reflects the patient's interests, with a minimum of personal bias.
- Communicate with nursing staff and consultants on a regular basis to convey critical information.
- Remain available to the patient and family for follow-up questions through all care transitions.
- Lead, coordinate or participate in hospital initiatives to assure adequate translator services and cross cultural sensitivities.

DIAGNOSTIC DECISION MAKING

Diagnostic decision making refers to the process of evaluating a patient complaint to develop a differential diagnosis, design a diagnostic evaluation, and arrive at a final diagnosis. Hospitalists frequently care for acutely ill patients with undifferentiated symptoms such as shortness of breath or chest pain. Establishing a correct diagnosis in these situations allows for timely therapeutic interventions and eliminates unnecessary diagnostic evaluation. Hospitalists assess disease prevalence, pre-test probability, and post-test probability to make a diagnostic decision. By using efficient and timely diagnostic decision making, hospitalists can positively impact the quality and cost of medical care.

KNOWLEDGE

Hospitalists should be able to:
- Describe the prevalence of common disease states to the local patient population.
- Explain appropriate resources to determine prevalence and incidence of disease states.
- Formulate a pretest probability using initial history, physical examination, and preliminary diagnostic information when available.
- Define and differentiate problem solving strategies, including hypothesis testing and pattern recognition.
- Define and differentiate prevalence, pre-test probability, test characteristics (including sensitivity, specificity, negative predictive value, positive predictive value, likelihood ratios), and post-test probability.
- Describe the concepts that underlie Bayes theorem, and how it is used in diagnostic decision making.
- Describe the relevance of sensitivity and specificity in interpreting diagnostic findings.
- Describe the sensitivity and specificity for common clinical syndromes of key clinical presentations and diagnostic findings.
- Name appropriate sources of information regarding evidence based clinical decision making.
- Describe the factors that account for excessive or indiscriminate testing.

SKILLS

Hospitalists should be able to:
- Obtain a targeted history, eliciting symptoms and data that help refine the diagnostic hypothesis.
- Perform a physical examination to further refine the diagnostic hypothesis.
- Order the indicated tests based on knowledge of disease prevalence, clinical uncertainty, and risk of morbidity and mortality.
- Calculate post-test probabilities of disease using pre-test probabilities and likelihood ratios.

ATTITUDES

Hospitalists should be able to:
- Communicate with patients and families to explain the differential diagnosis and evaluation of the patient's presenting symptoms.
- Communicate with patients and families to explain how testing will change the scope of diagnostic possibilities.
- Determine when sufficient evaluation has occurred, in the absence of diagnostic certainty.
- Communicate with other physicians, trainees and healthcare providers to explain the rationale for use of diagnostic tests.
- Recognize that each test should be preceded by a conscious decision to change or maintain the clinical care or initiate further diagnostic evaluation as indicated, based on the test results.
- Analyze the value of each diagnostic test, especially testing procedures that carry significant patient discomfort or risk.
- Appreciate that all tests have false positive and false negative results, and rigorously scrutinize or repeat the testing when the result is in question.
- Lead, coordinate or participate in the development of clinical care pathways.
- Incorporate the principles of evidenced based medicine, health care costs, and patient preferences and values into each patient's diagnostic evaluation.

DRUG SAFETY, PHARMACOECONOMICS AND PHARMACOEPIDEMIOLOGY

The number of new therapeutic agents approved by the Food and Drug Administration (FDA) is rapidly increasing. With the availability of these new agents and the widening use of other agents, pharmaceutical costs have grown more than any other sector of healthcare, as have concerns about adverse drug events (ADEs) from these agents. Hospitalists who strive to prescribe evidence based therapies must understand how to evaluate the benefits, harms, and financial costs of drug therapy for individual patients. Hospitalists promote and lead multidisciplinary teams to implement protocols, guidelines and clinical pathways that recommend preferred drug therapies. Hospitalists should be able to interpret outcomes measurement (pharmacoepidemiology) and economic analyses (pharmacoeconomics).

KNOWLEDGE

Hospitalists should be able to:
- Discuss principles of evaluating clinical efficacy, pharmacokinetics, dosing, drug and food interactions, and adverse effects that can affect the hospitalist's choice of agent, dosing frequency and route of administration.
- Explain options for measuring medication benefit.
- Explain the evidence based rationale for prophylactic drug therapies, comparing the costs, risks and benefits of competing strategies.
- Explain how pharmacodynamics change with age, liver disease and renal insufficiency.
- Describe the incidence of various types of ADEs in hospitalized patients, which may include adverse effects, interactions, and errors.
- Explain the role of polypharmacy in the development of delirium, ADEs, and noncompliance.
- Describe how the overuse of broad spectrum antibiotics promotes resistance.
- Describe key principles for interpreting pharmacoeconomic analyses including inflation rate, discounting rate, incremental analysis, sensitivity analysis, and inherent bias.
- Describe the clinical efficacy, safety profile, pharmacokinetics, dosing, drug and food interactions, and costs of commonly prescribed medications and biological agents (e.g., blood products).

SKILLS

Hospitalists should be able to:
- Prescribe medications for elderly hospitalized patients based on altered pharmacokinetics and co-morbid conditions.
- Apply treatment guidelines to individual patients in the use of antibiotics to reduce cost and the emergence of resistance.
- Minimize ADEs by using best practice models of medication ordering and administration.
- Document medications accurately and legibly taking into account approved abbreviation, and indicate start and stop dates for short-term medications.
- Arrange adequate follow-up for therapies that require outpatient monitoring, dosage adjustment, and education (e.g., anticoagulants, antibiotics).
- Balance the benefits, risks, and cost of prophylactic therapies, which may include venous thromboembolism and stress ulcer prophylaxis
- Convert intravenous medications to the oral route when indicated to promote patient safety, satisfaction, and reduce cost.
- Standardize blood transfusion practices.

ATTITUDES

Hospitalists should be able to:
- Educate patients and families about the importance of acquiring medication information and communicating medication history to clinicians at each transition of care.
- Ensure patients and families comprehend medication instructions.
- Recognize the benefits and hazards of drug therapy.
- Recognize the risk of ADEs at the time of transfer of care.

- Reconcile outpatient medications with inpatient medications at the time of admission and discharge.
- Reconcile all documentation of medications at the time of discharge.
- Integrate knowledge of benefits and risks of drug therapies into medical decision making for individual patients, and routinely reassess decisions.
- Critically assess and apply results of new outcome studies to improve drug treatment and patient safety for individual patients.
- Collaborate with pharmacists to improve drug safety for individual patients and reduce hospital costs.
- Apply the principles of pharmacoepidemiology and drug safety to patient management.
- Lead, coordinate and participate in the development, use, and dissemination of local, regional, and national practice guidelines and patient safety alerts pertaining to the prevention of complications.
- Apply the principles of pharmacoepidemiology and pharmacoeconomics to implement practice guidelines and protocols for a hospital.

EQUITABLE ALLOCATION OF RESOURCES

Health care expenditures in the United States continue to rise, reaching over $1.4 trillion in 2001 (14% of the gross domestic product), with hospital spending accounting for the largest portion. Hospitals are under constant pressure to provide more efficient care with limited resources. As hospitalists provide cost-effective inpatient care, they increasingly act as coordinators of care and resources in the hospital setting. Among the factors that make patients vulnerable to inequitable health care are race, ethnicity, and socioeconomic status. While disparity in care exists in United States hospitals, hospitalists are positioned to identify such disparities, optimize care for all patients, and advocate for equitable and cost-effective allocation of hospital resources.

KNOWLEDGE

Hospitalists should be able to:
- Define the concepts of equity and cost-effectiveness.
- Identify patient populations at risk for inequitable health care.
- Recognize health resources that are prone to inequitable allocations.
- Distinguish between decision analysis, cost-effectiveness analysis, and cost-benefit analysis.
- Explain how cost-effectiveness may conflict with equity in health care policies.
- Discuss how stereotypes impact the allocation of health resources.
- Demonstrate how equity in health care is cost effective.
- Illustrate how disparities in health care are related to quality of care.

SKILLS

Hospitalists should be able to:
- Measure patient access to hospital resources.
- Incorporate equity concerns into cost-effectiveness analysis.
- Triage patients to appropriate hospital resources.
- Construct cost-effective care pathways that allocate resources equitably.
- Monitor for equity in health care among hospitalized patients.
- Practice evidence based, cost-effective care for all patients.

ATTITUDES

Hospitalists should be able to:
- Listen to the concerns of all patients.
- Advocate for every patient's needed health services.
- Influence hospital policy to ensure equitable health care coverage for all hospitalized patients.
- Act on cultural differences or language barriers during patient encounters that may inhibit equality in health care.
- Recognize that over utilization of resources including excessive test ordering may not promote patient safety or patient satisfaction, or improve quality of care.
- Lead, coordinate or participate in multidisciplinary teams, which may include radiology, pharmacy, nursing and social services to decrease hospital costs and provide evidence based, cost effective care.
- Collaborate with information technologists and health care economists to track utilization and outcomes. Lead, coordinate or participate in quality improvement initiatives to improve resource allocation.
- Advocate using cost-effectiveness analysis, cost benefit analysis, evidence based medicine and measurements of health care equity to mold hospital policy on the allocation of its resources.
- Advocate for cross-cultural education and interpreter services into hospital systems to decrease barriers to equitable health care allocations.
- Lead, coordinate, or participate in multidisciplinary hospital and community efforts to ensure proper access to care for all individuals.

EVIDENCE BASED MEDICINE

Evidence based medicine (EBM) uses a systematic approach to medical decision making and patient care, combining the highest-available level of scientific evidence with practitioner clinical judgment and patient values and preferences. For hospitalists facing multiple critical medical choices daily, an EBM approach helps clinicians collaborate with patients to make the best possible decisions for their inpatient care. Hospitalists use study evidence to answer clinical questions and to develop quality improvement projects, including protocols and clinical pathways that can improve the efficiency, quality, and safety of care within their organizations. Hospitalists further provide leadership in educational efforts that foster a rigorous evidence based approach among medical trainees, hospital staff, and physician colleagues.

KNOWLEDGE

Hospitalists should be able to:
- Describe the necessary steps required to ask and answer clinical questions using standardized EBM methods.
- Describe the four core components of framing clinical questions using an EBM approach.
- Identify peer-reviewed databases and other resources to search for study evidence to answer clinical and systems questions.
- Differentiate between filtered and non-filtered resources, list examples of each, and describe the advantages and disadvantages of each.
- Describe major study types including therapy, diagnosis, prognosis, harm, meta-analysis (systematic review), economic analysis, and decision analysis.
- Describe and differentiate the important strengths and weaknesses of the following study designs: randomized controlled trials, meta-analyses, cohort studies, case-control studies, case series, cost-effectiveness studies, and clinical decision analysis studies.
- Explain the core components and core statistical concepts used in therapy studies, including relative risk, Relative Risk Reduction (RRR), Absolute Risk Reduction (ARR), Number Needed to Treat (NNT) and diagnosis studies, which may include sensitivity, specificity, and likelihood ratio.

SKILLS

Hospitalists should be able to:
- Formulate a well-designed clinical question using the Patient Intervention Comparison Outcome (PICO) approach.
- Identify the most appropriate study design(s) for the specific clinical or systems based question at hand.
- Search filtered and non-filtered information resources efficiently to find answers to clinical questions.
- Critically appraise the validity of individual study methodology and reporting.
- Evaluate and interpret study results, including useful point estimates and precision analysis.
- Apply relevant results of validated studies to individual patient care or systems improvement projects.

ATTITUDES

Hospitalists should be able to:
- Seek the best available evidence to support clinical decisions and process improvements at the individual and institutional level.
- Appreciate that filtered resources allow greater efficiency than non-filtered resources in searching for answers to clinical and systems questions and locating high-quality evidence.
- Reflect upon individual practice patterns to identify new questions.
- Develop a process for the ongoing incorporation of new information into existing clinical practice and system improvement projects.
- Serve as a role model for evidence based point-of-care practice.
- Influence and support other clinicians to develop and utilize EBM skills to improve clinical practice and systems or processes within practice.
- Lead, coordinate or participate in systems interventions to improve the quality, efficiency and standardization of care based on EBM review of the literature.
- Advocate for the institution to provide or facilitate access to high quality point-of-care EBM information resources.

HOSPITALIST AS CONSULTANT

Hospitalists may provide expert medical opinion regarding the care of hospitalized patients or may serve as consultants for patients under the care of other medical and surgical services. The hospitalist consultant may provide opinions and recommendations or actively manage the patient's hospital care. Effective and frequent communication between the hospitalist and the requesting physician ensures safe and quality care. Hospitalists should promote communication between services to improve the care of the hospitalized patient, optimize resource utilization, and enhance patient safety.

KNOWLEDGE

Hospitalists should be able to:
- Define the role of the hospitalist consultant.
- Describe the components of an effective consultation.
- Assess the urgency of the consultation and the questions posed by the requesting physician.
- List factors that may affect implementation of consultant's recommendations.

SKILLS

Hospitalists should be able to:
- Obtain a thorough and relevant history and review the medical record.
- Perform a relevant physical examination.
- Interpret indicated diagnostic studies.
- Synthesize a treatment plan based on the data obtained from the history, physical examination and diagnostic studies.
- Summarize the findings in the patient record.
- List concise but specific recommendations for management.
- Communicate recommendations to the consulting physician in an expedient and efficient manner.
- Assess the level of care required, and communicate with the requesting physician if a transition of care is advised.

ATTITUDES

Hospitalists should be able to:
- Determine the hospitalist consultant's role in collaboration with the requesting physician.
- Respond promptly to the requesting physician's need for consultation.
- Lead by example by performing consultations in a collegial, professional and non-confrontational manner.
- Inform and educate the requesting physician of potential complications and opportunities for prevention of complications.
- Provide frequent follow-up, including review of pertinent findings and laboratory data, and ensure that critical recommendations have been followed.
- Provide timely and effective communication with the requesting physician/team.
- Transmit written communication legibly and with clear contact information.
- Recognize when the hospitalist's role in the patient's care is complete, document final recommendations in the medical record, and maintain availability.
- Communicate with patient and family to convey recommendations and treatment plans.
- Recognize the importance of arranging appropriate follow-up.
- Lead, coordinate or participate in multidisciplinary initiatives to promote patient safety and optimize resource utilization.

HOSPITALIST AS TEACHER

Hospitalist as teacher refers to specific interactions with members of the multidisciplinary care team to educate them about inpatient care plans, hospital protocols, patient safety, and evidence based clinical problem solving. As educators, hospitalists provide leadership in patient care, teach at multiple levels, and facilitate team building. Hospitalists serve as role models and teach the process of clinical decision making as a tool for future physician-patient encounters. Hospitalists may review, modify, and promote new protocols and guidelines to implement across multiple services in the hospital. The hospitalist as teacher is a core competency essential to the process of effecting organizational change.

KNOWLEDGE

Hospitalists should be able to:
- Describe adult education principles.
- Explain the conditions that facilitate and inhibit learning.
- Define the concept of a teachable moment.
- Describe the process of developing a formal educational session, which may include needs assessment, determining goals and objectives, development of materials and teaching activities, and evaluation
- Describe practical steps that may be taken to deliver dynamic presentations for multiple venues, which may include bedside teaching to trainees, small group discussions with co-workers or managers, academic detailing for new initiatives, and didactic lectures at national meetings.
- Describe teaching microskills, including obtaining a commitment, probing for supporting evidence, teaching general rules, reinforcing what was right, and correcting mistakes.
- Describe the benefits and limitations of various teaching modalities.
- Identify resources for training materials.
- Explain how the SHM Core Competencies can be applied to curricular development.
- Explain the role of the hospitalist as a teacher.

SKILLS

Hospitalists should be able to:
- Establish a comfortable and safe learning environment.
- Establish expectations for each teaching session and clearly articulate the objectives.
- Effectively communicate the goals of the learning session and assess progress towards those goals.
- Instruct at the level of learner experience and knowledge, and accommodate for learners at different levels.
- Determine the information needs of the intended recipient and evaluate performance.
- Tailor messages to the needs and abilities of intended recipient.
- Structure and organize the timing and delivery of information and learning experiences to maximize comprehension.
- Utilize adult learning principles in the development or selection of educational programs, methods and materials.
- Use explicit and relevant language to explain clinical reasoning process for the learner, who may include patients and families.
- Make the clinical reasoning process understandable, explicit, and relevant.
- Promote clinical problem solving during each patient encounter.
- Provide bedside teaching that is informative and comfortable for patients, trainees and members of the multidisciplinary care team.
- Demonstrate effective mentoring, which may include role modeling.
- Demonstrate procedures by explaining indications and contraindications, equipment, each sequential step in the procedure, and necessary follow-up.
- Demonstrate an efficient and succinct approach to clinical care.
- Provide prompt, explicit, and action-oriented feedback.

ATTITUDES

Hospitalists should be able to:

- Advocate the importance of lifelong learning and mentorship.
- Balance patient care and teaching.
- Demonstrate concern for the privacy and dignity of the patient.
- Adhere to time constraints.
- Establish a trusting relationship with patients and families, medical trainees, and the multidisciplinary team.
- Demonstrate respect for all learners at various knowledge and skill levels.
- Promote evaluation standards that are fair and prompt and facilitate career development.
- Appreciate the needs of the learner and the patient.
- Project enthusiasm for the teaching role.
- Admit the limitations of one's knowledge and respond appropriately to mistakes.
- Encourage and provide the tools for life-long, self-directed learning and clinical problem solving.
- Lead, coordinate or participate in efforts to formulate a needs assessment program for hospitalists' continued professional development.
- Lead, coordinate and participate in educational scholarship.
- Seek feedback on the effectiveness of instruction methods, modalities and materials.
- Reflect on teaching moments to identify opportunities for improvement.
- Promote evidence based information acquisition and clinical decision making.
- Utilize the role of the hospitalist as a clinician educator to lead, coordinate or participate in quality improvement initiatives.

INFORMATION MANAGEMENT

Information management refers to the acquisition and utilization of patient data for key hospital activities that include but are not limited to direct patient care. Optimal care of hospitalized patients and optimal work flow require basic clinical information systems. Advanced clinical information systems also provide decision support, which may include computer based provider order entry, event monitoring, electronic charting and bar coding. Hospitalists use local systems to acquire data and information that support optimal medical decision making at the point of care. Hospitalists can lead or coordinate efforts within their institution to develop, utilize and update clinical information systems to improve patient outcomes, reduce costs, and increase satisfaction among providers.

KNOWLEDGE

Hospitalists should be able to:
- Describe how hospital information systems are utilized by different departments to manage patient registration and financial data, process clinical results, and schedule appointments and tests.
- Identify and describe how to access available sources of reference information, which may include literature search engines, online textbooks, electronic calculators and practice guidelines to support optimal patient care.
- Explain how information systems can facilitate the practice of evidence based medical decision making.
- Explain how computer physician order entry (CPOE) with decision support favorably impacts on patient safety in the hospital setting.
- Explain potential pitfalls of the use of CPOE.
- Describe potential advantages and disadvantages of written and electronic patient records.
- Explain the limitations of different forms of data and data systems available to clinicians and how information systems can facilitate timely and accurate clinician submissions of bills.
- Explain Health Insurance Portability and Accountability Act (HIPAA) regulations and their impact on management of patient information.

SKILLS

Hospitalists should be able to:
- Efficiently retrieve and interpret data, images, and other information from available clinical information systems.
- Interpret data from digital devices, which may include EKG monitors, glucometers, or oxygen saturation monitors.
- Access and interpret information from internet-based clinical information systems when available.
- Interpret results incorporating statistical principles of probability and uncertainty.

ATTITUDES

Hospitalists should be able to:
- Recognize the limitations of acquisition devices or equipment, and use clinical judgment to interpret results that fall either within or outside the expected ranges.
- Recognize the influence of individual patient factors in the interpretation of available information.
- Adhere to principles of data integrity, security and confidentiality.
- Lead, coordinate or participate in multidisciplinary initiatives to adopt hospital information systems that improve efficiency and optimize patient care.
- Lead, coordinate or participate in multidisciplinary initiatives to continuously improve hospital information systems and physician practice patterns by providing constructive feedback and advice in system development.
- Advocate for order entry systems that promote patient safety and ease of use.
- Advocate for information decision support to facilitate efficient and optimal medical management.
- Identify issues, provide feedback, and resolve conflicts within an information systems framework.

LEADERSHIP

Hospitalists assume formal and informal leadership roles in the hospital system and community. In their individual institutions, hospitalists are responsible for the management and coordination of patient care. This role requires advocating for the patient, building consensus, and balancing the needs of individual patients with the resources available to the hospital. Hospitalists also lead efforts to assess, identify and improve patient outcomes, resource utilization, cost-effectiveness, and quality of inpatient medical care. In the larger community, hospitalists lead innovations in hospital medicine research and education and the delivery of health care.

KNOWLEDGE

Hospitalists should be able to:
- Differentiate management and leadership.
- Describe hospitalist responsibilities and opportunities to provide active leadership.
- Describe the key elements of a message.
- Discuss how mentor relationships impact the development and advancement of the field of hospital medicine.
- Explain the attributes and effects of modeling positive and negative behaviors.
- Name the key elements of strategic planning processes.
- Explain factors that predict the success or failure of strategic plans.
- Describe styles of leadership.
- Explain the attributes of effective leadership.
- Articulate the business and financial motivators that impact decision making.
- Explain the specific factors that affect positive change.
- Explain effective negotiation and conflict resolution techniques.

SKILLS

Hospitalists should be able to:
- Tailor messages to specific target audiences.
- Develop effective communication skills using multiple modalities.
- Plan and conduct an effective meeting.
- Construct program mission and vision statements.
- Develop personal, team and program goals, and identify indicators of achievement.
- Establish, measure and report key performance metrics.
- Utilize established metrics to assess progress and set new goals for performance and outcomes.
- Analyze personal leadership style.
- Demonstrate the ability to effectively work with various leadership styles.
- Develop budgets to support goals using accepted financial principles.
- Translate performance into measurable financial outcomes.
- Assess the barriers and facilitating factors to effect change and incorporate those factors into a strategic approach.
- Demonstrate effective and creative problem solving techniques.
- Resolve conflicts using specific negotiation techniques.

ATTITUDES

Hospitalists should be able to:
- Lead by example.
- Practice active listening techniques.
- Provide and seek timely, useful feedback.
- Provide leadership in teaching, educational scholarship, quality improvement and other areas that serve to improve patient outcomes and advance the field of hospital medicine.
- Explain the importance of finding mentor(s) and serving as a mentor.
- Recognize the importance and influence of positive role modeling.

- Assess and address personal leadership strengths and weaknesses.
- Seek and participate in opportunities for professional development.
- Advocate for financial and other resources needed to support goals and initiatives.
- Exemplify professionalism.
- Accept responsibility and accountability for management decisions.
- Build consensus in support of key decisions.

MANAGEMENT PRACTICES

Management practice in hospital medicine refers to program/medical group development and growth, practice management, contract negotiation, performance measurement and financial analysis. Hospitalists require fundamental management skills to enhance their individual success, and to facilitate growth and stability of their hospital medicine groups and institutions in which they practice. Hospitals increasingly need physician leaders with management skills to improve operational efficiency and meet other institutional needs. Hospitalists must acquire and maintain management skills that allow them to define their role and value, create a strategic plan for practice growth, anticipate and respond to change, and achieve financial success.

KNOWLEDGE

Hospitalists should be able to:
- Describe different models of physician compensation and incentives.
- Explain the impact of third-party payer contracts on hospital reimbursement.
- Discuss the potential impact of Pay for Performance initiatives on patient care, and expectations for individual hospitalists and hospital medicine groups.
- Describe Federal statutory restrictions on physicians contracting with hospitals, third-party payers and group practices.
- Describe the impact of medication formularies, utilization review requirements, third party payer contracts and other policies impacting patient care.
- Describe required system improvements needed to meet new healthcare legislation or public health guidelines.
- Describe the personnel file, its contents and usage.
- Define the role and value of hospitalists and hospital medicine programs.
- Explain advantages and disadvantages of utilizing physician extenders in a hospital medicine practice.
- Describe the necessary elements for effective and compliant billing, coding, and revenue capture.
- Define commonly used hospital financial terminology, including but not limited to procedure codes, relative value units (RVUs), direct and indirect costs, average length of stay, and case mix index.
- Define the components of a useful financial report.

SKILLS

Hospitalists should be able to:
- Apply basic accounting practices to track financial performance and develop a practice budget.
- Develop practice staffing arrangements and schedules.
- Market the hospital medicine program.
- Develop job descriptions for physician and non-physician employees to facilitate accountability and professional development.
- Develop strategies for recruiting and retaining hospitalists.
- Conduct or participate in performance reviews for physician and non-physician staff.
- Negotiate effectively with physicians, medical practices, hospitals, and third party payers.
- Interpret hospital generated reports on individual and group performance.
- Assess satisfaction of community physicians, patients, nurses and other user groups.
- Develop strategic planning processes to meet individual and group goals and establish accountability.
- Develop business plans to facilitate growth of the practice.
- Prepare an annual review of program performance for the hospital executive team.
- Demonstrate teamwork, organization, and leadership skills.

ATTITUDES

Hospitalists should be able to:
- Lead by example.
- Recognize the importance of routine critical analysis of all aspects of practice operations to optimize efficiency, quality and efficacy.
- Recognize the importance of meeting or exceeding customer and colleague expectations.
- Recognize the importance of best management practice.
- Recognize the importance of marketing and public relations to foster sustainable practice growth.

NUTRITION AND THE HOSPITALIZED PATIENT

Optimal nutrition in the hospital can facilitate better patient outcomes. Malnutrition in hospitalized patients can lead to poor wound healing, impaired immune function resulting in infectious complications, increased hospital length of stay, and overall increased morbidity and mortality. The prevalence of malnutrition has been reported in up to 50% of hospitalized patients. Early screening for nutritional risk allows for appropriate intervention in the hospital setting, as well as planning for appropriate home services and follow-up for outpatient nutritional care. Hospitalists use a multidisciplinary approach to evaluate and address the nutritional needs of hospitalized patients. Hospitalists lead, coordinate or participate in multidisciplinary initiatives to improve the nutritional status of hospitalized patients.

KNOWLEDGE

Hospitalists should be able to:
- Describe methods of screening for malnutrition.
- Identify when a nutrition evaluation by a registered dietitian is required.
- Differentiate between basic modified diets and explain the indications for each (sodium, diabetic, renal, and different dietary consistencies).
- Explain the indications and contraindications for enteral nutrition.
- Describe the indications for parenteral nutrition.
- Describe potential complications associated with enteral and parenteral nutrition.
- Explain risk factors for the re-feeding syndrome.

SKILLS

Hospitalists should be able to:
- Use objective criteria to determine if a patient is malnourished.
- Determine appropriate laboratory measures to ascertain presence of malnutrition.
- Utilize individualized modified diets and/or nutritional supplements, which may include total parenteral nutrition, based on the patient's medical condition.
- Choose an appropriate enteral nutrition formula when indicated.
- Treat for electrolyte abnormalities associated with the re-feeding syndrome.
- Monitor electrolytes as indicated in the setting of enteral and/or parenteral nutritional support.

ATTITUDES

Hospitalists should be able to:
- Recognize the importance of adequate nutrition in hospitalized patients.
- Recognize when a nutrition evaluation by a registered dietitian is required.
- Consult a nutrition specialist for a comprehensive nutritional evaluation when indicated.
- Collaborate with clinical nutrition staff to implement the nutrition care plan.
- Utilize a team approach for early discharge planning for patients requiring home parenteral or enteral nutrition.
- Recognize that specialized nutritional supplementation may be required in certain patient populations, which may include patients with extensive wounds or increased catabolic needs.
- Implement routine nutrition screening to identify malnourished patients early in admission.
- Lead, coordinate or participate in the development of care pathways for patients requiring enteral or parenteral nutrition.
- Coordinate follow-up nutrition care as part of discharge plans for those patients requiring nutritional support.

PALLIATIVE CARE

Palliative care refers to a collaborative, comprehensive, interdisciplinary approach to improve the quality of life of patients living with debilitating, chronic or terminal illness. Palliative care is appropriate at any stage of illness and should be provided simultaneously with all other medical treatments. This approach includes the prevention and relief of suffering by means of early identification, assessment, and treatment of pain and other distressing symptoms such as dyspnea, nausea, fatigue, anxiety and depression; and attention to the physical, psychosocial and spiritual needs of patients and their families.

Hospitalists provide palliative care in multiple realms including 1) patients dying in the hospital; 2) patients discharged to home or another institution for end-of-life care; 3) patients with newly diagnosed life-threatening illness; 4) patients requiring complex inpatient symptom management interventions; 5) patients for whom it is appropriate to shift the goal of care away from disease cure or stabilization and toward the maximization of comfort; and 6) patients with serious, chronic illness such as heart failure, COPD, liver disease, dementia, and cancer. Hospitalists lead, coordinate, and participate in initiatives to improve the identification and treatment of patients and families in need of palliative care.

KNOWLEDGE

Hospitalists should be able to:
- Determine effective management strategies for patients requiring palliative care.
- Describe potential adverse effects from medications and procedures directed at palliation.
- Formulate strategies for prevention and treatment of complications of palliative care interventions.
- Assess the impact of interventions including feeding tubes, parenteral nutrition, mechanical ventilation, and intravenous fluids on patient comfort and prognosis.
- Describe the concept of "double effect" with respect to palliative care intervention.
- Name the basic tenets of hospice care and the Medicare hospice benefit.
- Identify indicators of clinical stability that allow for safe transitions of care and continuity after discharge.
- Explain the role of palliative care throughout the course of illness and how it can be provided alongside all other appropriate medical treatments.
- Describe signs and symptoms of the last 24 hours of life and how to discuss these observations with families.
- Describe the responsibilities of the hospitalist after a patient dies, including pronouncing a person dead, completing the death certificate, requesting an autopsy, notifying family and PCP, and contacting the organ donor network.

SKILLS

Hospitalists should be able to:
- Obtain a thorough and relevant history, review the medical record, and perform a comprehensive physical examination to identify symptoms, co-morbidities, medications or social influences that impact the palliative care plan.
- Direct individual patient's palliative care delivery from admission to discharge.
- Formulate a communication plan for delivering prognostic information.
- Conduct effective and compassionate family meetings.
- Formulate specific patient centered palliative care plans that include pain management; integration of psychiatric, social, spiritual and other support services; and discharge planning.
- Recognize and address the psychosocial effects of complex, acute life threatening illness in hospitalized patients.
- Assess and respond to patient's symptoms, which may include pain, dyspnea, nausea, constipation, fatigue, anorexia, anxiety, depression and delirium.
- Anticipate adverse effects and "double effect" from interventions and initiate measures to minimize such problems.
- Communicate effectively with patients and families about patient's values and goals of care.
- Communicate effectively with patients and families about hospice and know how to refer a patient to hospice.
- Respond to patient requests for assisted suicide and identify and address other important ethical issues.

ATTITUDES

Hospitalists should be able to:

- Convey diagnosis, prognosis, treatment and support options available for patients and families in a clear, concise, compassionate, culturally sensitive and timely manner.
- Determine patient and family understanding of severity of illness, prognosis and their role in determining the goals of their care.
- Promote the ethical imperative of frequent pain assessment and adequate control.
- Appreciate that all pain is subjective and acknowledge patient's self reports of pain.
- Discuss with patients and families goals for pain management strategies and functional status and set targets for pain control.
- Appreciate that good palliative care for patients with certain conditions often involves the use of therapies typically thought of as curative.
- Conduct meetings with patients and families to establish goals of care that reflect the patient's wishes.
- Determine existence of advance directives and provide patients and families with resources to understand and execute such directives.
- Advocate incorporation of patient wishes into care plans.
- Recognize the need for frequent family meetings.
- Address resuscitation status and patient preferences for care early during hospital stay.
- Maintain rapport with patients and families and a consistent approach to management during transfers of care.
- Recognize impact of cultural and spiritual factors to the provision of palliative care.
- Appreciate the role of other members of the healthcare team including nursing and social services, pharmacy, psychology and pastoral care in providing comprehensive palliative care, and work closely with these team members in caring for patients with serious, chronic and terminal illnesses and their families.
- Provide reassurance to patients and families that clinical providers will be available to provide ongoing care and relief of symptoms.
- Formulate a comprehensive discharge plan that will empower the patient, family and subsequent providers to anticipate and manage changing symptoms, emergency situations, and increasing dependency.
- Lead, coordinate or participate in efforts to establish or improve palliative care in the hospital, which may include establishing a palliative care consultation service.
- Consider palliative care issues at hospital management and committee meetings.
- Engage providers and administrators in the study of local palliative care delivery to include efficacy of pain assessment and intervention, patient and family satisfaction with care delivery, impact on hospital occupancy and costs, and fulfilled expectations of referring and collaborating providers and services.

PATIENT EDUCATION

The Institute of Medicine has defined patient centered care as one of the six aims for healthcare improvements in the 21st century. Patient centered care requires that physicians and members of multidisciplinary teams effectively inform, educate, reassure and empower patients and families to participate in the creation and implementation of a care plan. Patient safety initiatives focus on the role of patient education in improving the quality of care from the perspective of both patients and clinicians. Hospitalists can develop and promote strategies to improve patient education initiatives and foster greater patient and family involvement in health care decisions and management.

KNOWLEDGE

Hospitalists should be able to:
- Describe the guiding principles for patient education.
- Explain the factors that impact the success or failure of behavior change strategies.
- Identify institutional resources for patient education materials and programs.
- Summarize the evidence for the primacy of patient education as a means to improve the quality of health care.
- Discuss the contextual factors that influence a patient's readiness to learn new information.
- Describe the role of patient education in the management of chronic diseases, which may include diabetes, congestive heart failure, and asthma.
- Explain how each patient's socio-cultural background affects his or her health beliefs and behavior.
- Identify barriers to implementation of patient education, including literacy levels and language fluency.
- Determine the utility and appropriateness of patient education materials based on specific patient characteristics, which may include culture, literacy, cognitive ability, age, native language, and visual or other sensory impairments.

SKILLS

Hospitalists should be able to:
- Identify and assist patients and families who require additional education about their medical illnesses.
- Communicate effectively with patients from diverse backgrounds.
- Formulate specific patient centered care plans that may include pain management; integration of psychiatric, social, and other support services; and discharge planning.
- Describe different methods of delivering patient education and effectively apply this knowledge to the care of individual patients.
- Utilize and/or develop methods and materials to fully inform patients and families.
- Determine patient and family understanding of severity of illness, prognosis, and their role in determining the goals of care.
- Provide patients with safety tips at the time of transfer of care, which may include instructions about medications, tests, procedures, alert symptoms to initiate a physician call, and follow-up.

ATTITUDES

Hospitalists should be able to:
- Recognize the potential for patient education to improve the quality of health care.
- Encourage patients to ask questions, keep accurate medication lists and obtain test results.
- Ensure that patients understand anticipated therapies, procedures and/or surgery.
- Convey diagnosis, prognosis, treatment and support options available for patients and families in a clear, concise, compassionate, culturally sensitive and timely manner.
- Provide or arrange for patient education materials and programs for patients with chronic diseases.
- Advocate incorporation of patient wishes into care plans.
- Appreciate patient education as a tool to improve the experience of clinical care for both patients and families.
- Lead, coordinate or participate in the development of team-based approaches to patient education.
- Lead, coordinate or participate in the development of effective quality measures sensitive to the effects of patient education.

PATIENT HANDOFF

Patient handoff (or sign-out) refers to the specific interaction, communication, and planning required to achieve seamless transitions of care from one clinician to another. Effective and timely sign-outs are essential to maintain high quality medical care, reduce medical errors and redundancy, and prevent loss of information. Hospitalists are involved in the transfer of patient care on a daily basis and can lead institutional initiatives that promote optimal transfer of information between health care providers.

KNOWLEDGE

Hospitalists should be able to:
- Describe key elements involved in signing out a patient.
- Explain important information that should be communicated during patient sign-out, which may include administrative details, updated clinical status, tasks to be completed and relative priority, severity of illness assessment, code status, and contingency planning.
- Explain the components and strategies that are critical for successful communication during sign-outs.
- Explain how the components, strategies and specific information provided at sign-out might vary depending on complexity of the patient, familiarity of provider with the patient and the care environment, and timing of sign-out.
- Explain the strengths and limitations of various sign-out communication strategies and procedures.

SKILLS

Hospitalists should be able to:
- Communicate effectively and efficiently during patient sign-out.
- Demonstrate the use of read back when communicating tasks.
- Utilize the most efficient and effective verbal and written communication modalities.
- Construct patient summaries for oral and written delivery, incorporating the unique characteristics of the patient, provider and timing of the sign-out.
- Evaluate all medications for indication, dosing, and planned duration at the time of sign-out.
- Document updated clinical status, recent and pending test and study results, a complete problem list, and plans for continued care.
- Explain the importance of using "if-then" statements for critical tasks to be completed.
- Anticipate what may go wrong with a patient after a transition in care and communicate this clearly to the receiving clinician.
- Synthesize medical information received from Hospitalists signing out patients into care plans

ATTITUDES

Hospitalists should be able to:
- Inform patients and families in advance of sign-out.
- Recognize the impact of effective and ineffective sign-outs on patient safety.
- Appreciate the value of *real time* interactive dialogue between hospitalists during sign-out.
- Review received sign-out summaries and communications information carefully and request clarification when needed.
- Engage stakeholders in hospital initiatives to continuously assess the quality of sign-outs.
- Lead, coordinate or participate in initiatives to develop and implement new protocols to improve and optimize sign-outs.
- Lead, coordinate or participate in evaluation of new strategies or information systems designed to improve sign-outs.
- Promote availability after sign-outs should questions arise.

PATIENT SAFETY

The National Patient Safety Foundation defines safety as the avoidance, prevention and amelioration of adverse outcomes or injuries stemming from the processes of health care. Hospitalized patients are at risk for a variety of adverse events. Hospitalists anticipate complications from medical assessment and treatment, and take steps to reduce their incidence or severity. Application of individual and system failure analysis can improve patient safety. Hospitalists will increasingly lead and participate in multidisciplinary development of interventions to mitigate system and process failures. They will also need to assess the effects of recommended interventions across the continuum of care.

KNOWLEDGE

Hospitalists should be able to:
- Identify the most common safety problems and their causes in different hospitalized patient populations.
- Explain the role of human factors in device, procedure and technology-related errors.
- Specify clinical practices and interventions that improve the safe use of high-alert medications.
- Summarize methods of system and process evaluation of patient safety.
- Describe the elements of well-functioning teams.
- Differentiate retrospective and prospective methods of evaluating medical errors.
- Discuss the significance of sentinel events and "near misses" and their relationship to voluntary and mandatory reporting regulations.
- Describe the components of Root Cause Analysis (RCA) and Failure Mode and Effects Analysis (FMEA).

SKILLS

Hospitalists should be able to:
- Prevent iatrogenic complications and proactively reduce risks of hospitalization.
- Formulate age- and disease-specific safety practices, which may include reduction of incidence and severity of falls, decubitus ulcers, delirium, hospital-acquired infections, venous thromboembolism, malnutrition, and medication adverse events.
- Develop, implement and evaluate practice guidelines and care pathways as part of an interdisciplinary quality improvement initiative.
- Gather, record and transfer patient information utilizing timely, accurate and confidential mechanisms.
- Develop systems that promote patient safety and reduce the likelihood of adverse events.
- Contribute to and interpret retrospective RCA and prospective Healthcare FMEA multidisciplinary risk evaluations.
- Function as a member and/or leader of interdisciplinary safety teams.
- Design evaluation methods and resources to define problems and recommend interventions.

ATTITUDES

Hospitalists should be able to:
- Appreciate that adverse drug events must be monitored and steps taken to reduce their incidence.
- Advocate and help foster a non-punitive error-reporting environment.
- Exemplify safe medication prescribing and administration practices.
- Facilitate practices that reduce the likelihood of hospital-acquired infection.
- Internalize and promote behaviors that minimize workforce fatigue, occupational illness and burnout.
- Appreciate that redundant systems may reduce the likelihood of medical errors.
- Understand the risk management issues of patient safety efforts.
- Utilize evidence based evaluation methods and resources when defining problems and designing interventions.
- Lead, coordinate or participate in multidisciplinary teams to improve the delivery of safe patient care.
- Judge the effect of patient volume on the quality, efficiency and safety of healthcare services.
- Prioritize patient safety evaluation and improvement efforts based on the impact, improvability and general applicability of proposed evaluations and interventions.

- Employ continuous quality improvement techniques to identify, construct, implement and evaluate patient safety issues.
- Lead, coordinate or participate in the development, use and dissemination of local, regional, or national clinical practice guidelines and patient safety alerts pertaining to the prevention of complications in hospitalized patients.
- Lead, coordinate or participate in efforts to create a culture in which issues of patient safety and medical errors can be discussed openly, without fear of repercussion.

PRACTICE BASED LEARNING AND IMPROVEMENT

Practice Based Learning and Improvement (PBLI) is a means of evaluating individual and system practice patterns and incorporating the best available evidence to improve patient care. PBLI is recognized as a critical skill for all clinicians by the Accreditation Council for Graduate Medical Education (ACGME), the American Board of Internal Medicine (ABIM), and the American Board of Pediatrics (ABP). As the practice of Hospital Medicine rapidly evolves, hospitalists apply the most up-to-date knowledge to their care of inpatients. Hospitalists use a PBLI approach to lead, coordinate and participate in initiatives to improve hospital processes and clinical care.

KNOWLEDGE

Hospitalists should be able to:
- Describe systematic methods of analyzing practice experience.
- Explain key concepts of practice based improvement methodology, which include the Plan Do Study Act (PDSA) model.
- Define the role of multidisciplinary teams and team leaders in improving patient care.
- Describe how critical appraisal skills, including study design, statistical methods and clinical relevance apply to PBLI.
- Describe how information technology can be used to identify opportunities to improve patient care.

SKILLS

Hospitalists should be able to:
- Translate information about a general population into management of subpopulations or individual patients.
- Critically assess individual and system practice patterns and experience to identify areas for improvement and minimize heterogeneity of practice.
- Design practice interventions to improve quality, efficiency, and consistency of patient care using standard PBLI methodology and tools.
- Assess medical information to support self-directed learning.
- Establish and maintain an open dialogue with patients and families regarding care goals and limitations, palliative care, and end of life issues.
- Critically appraise and apply the reports of new medical evidence.
- Use health information systems efficiently to manage and improve care at the individual and system levels.
- Utilize evidence based information resources to inform clinical decisions.

ATTITUDES

Hospitalists should be able to:
- Advocate for the use of PBLI in clinical practice and in system improvement projects.
- Create an environment conducive to self-evaluation and improvement.
- Advocate for investment in information technology.
- Facilitate and encourage self-directed learning among health care professionals and trainees.
- Promote self improvement and care standardization, utilizing best evidence and practice.

PREVENTION OF HEALTHCARE-ASSOCIATED INFECTIONS
AND ANTIMICROBIAL RESISTANCE

Healthcare-associated infections impose a significant burden on the healthcare system in the Unites States, both economically and in terms of patient outcomes. The Centers for Disease Control and Prevention (CDC) estimate that nearly 2 million patients develop healthcare-associated infections each year, and approximately 88,000 die as a direct or indirect result of their infections. These infections often lead to increases in length of hospitalization, and result in about $4.5 billion in excess costs annually. The central aim of infection control is to prevent healthcare-associated infections and the emergence of resistant organisms. Hospitalists work in concert with other members of the healthcare organization to reduce healthcare-associated infections, develop institutional initiatives for prevention, and promote and implement evidence based infection control measures.

KNOWLEDGE

Hospitalists should be able to:

- Describe acceptable methods of hand hygiene technique and timing in relationship to patient contact.
- Describe the prophylactic measures required for all types of isolation precautions, which include Standard, Contact, Droplet, and Airborne Precautions, and list the indications for implementing each type of precaution.
- List common types of healthcare-associated infections, and describe the risk factors associated with urinary tract infections, surgical site infections, hospital-acquired pneumonia, and blood stream infections.
- Explain the utility of the hospital antibiogram in delineating antimicrobial resistance patterns for bacterial isolates, and how it should be used to make empiric antibiotic selections.
- Identify major resources for infection control information, including hospital infection control staff, hospital infection control policies and procedures, local and state public health departments, and CDCP guidelines.
- Describe the indicated prevention measures necessary to perform hospital-based procedures in a sterile fashion.

SKILLS

Hospitalists should be able to:

- Perform consistent and optimal hand hygiene techniques at all indicated points of care.
- Implement indicated isolation precautions for patients with high risk transmissible diseases or highly resistant infections.
- Identify and utilize local hospital resources, including antibiograms and infection control officers.
- Perform indicated infection control and prevention technique during all procedures.
- Implement precautions and infection control practices to protect patients from acquiring healthcare-associated infections.

ATTITUDES

Hospitalists should be able to:

- Appreciate that specific infection control practices and engineering controls are required to protect very high risk patient populations, which may include hematopoietic stem cell transplant or solid organ transplant recipients, from healthcare associated infections.
- Serve as a role model in adherence to recommended hand hygiene and infection control practices.
- Communicate effectively the rationale and importance of infection control practices to patients, families, visitors, other health care providers and hospital staff.
- Communicate appropriate patient information to infection control staff regarding potentially transmissible diseases.
- Avoid devices that are more likely to cause hospital-acquired infections if alternatives are safe, effective and available.
- Encourage removal of invasive devices, especially central venous catheters and urinary catheters, early during hospital stay and as soon as clinically safe to do so.
- Collaborate with multidisciplinary teams, which may include infection control, nursing service, and infectious disease consultants, to rapidly implement and maintain isolation precautions.

- Collaborate with multidisciplinary teams that may include infection control, nursing service, care coordination, long term care facilities, home health care staff, and public health personnel to plan for hospital discharge of patients with transmissible infectious diseases.
- Lead, coordinate or participate in efforts to educate other health care personnel and hospital staff about necessary infection control prevention measures.
- Lead, coordinate or participate in multidisciplinary teams that organize, implement, and study infection control protocols, guidelines or pathways, using evidence based systematic methods.
- Lead, coordinate or participate in multidisciplinary efforts to develop empiric antibiotic regimens to minimize the development of resistance within a particular hospital or region.

PROFESSIONALISM AND MEDICAL ETHICS

Professionalism refers to guidelines and attributes that require the physician to serve the interests of the patient above his or her self-interest. At the individual practitioner level, this denotes a commitment to the highest standards of excellence in the practice of medicine and in the generation and dissemination of knowledge to sustain the interests and welfare of patients. Within the practice of hospital medicine, professionalism also includes a commitment to be responsive to the health needs of society and a commitment to ethical principles. Hospitalists frequently encounter ethical dilemmas in their daily practice because issues arise regarding end of life care, the ability of the patient to consent to treatment, and pressures of resource utilization. Hospitalists lead, coordinate and participate in systems improvements that promote professionalism in health care delivery.

KNOWLEDGE

Hospitalists should be able to:
- Define and differentiate ethical principles, which may include beneficence and nonmaleficence, justice, patient autonomy, truth-telling, informed consent, and confidentiality.
- Describe the concept of double effect.
- Define and differentiate competency and decision making capacity.
- Explain the utility of power of attorney and advance directives in medical care.
- List the key elements of informed consent.
- Explain determination of decision making capacity and steps required for surrogate decision making.
- Describe local laws and regulations relevant to the practice of hospital medicine.
- Explain medical futility.

SKILLS

Hospitalists should be able to:
- Observe doctor-patient confidentiality and identify family members or surrogates to whom information can be released.
- Communicate with patient and family members on a regular basis.
- Recommend treatment options that optimize patient care, include consideration of resource utilization, and are formulated without regard to financial incentives or other conflicts of interest.
- Evaluate patients for medical decision making capacity.
- Obtain informed consent when indicated.
- Review power of attorney and advanced directives with patients and family members.
- Provide compassionate and relevant end of life care.
- Apply ethical principles to inpatient care.
- Follow patient's wishes as described by the patient, as outlined in advanced directives, or as described by the patient's surrogate decision maker.

ATTITUDES

Hospitalists should be able to:
- Commit to life-long self learning, maintenance of skills, and clinical excellence.
- Promote access to medical care for the community.
- Recognize when consultation from others who have expertise in psychiatry and ethics will promote optimal care for patients and help resolve ethical dilemmas.
- Provide compassionate and relevant care for patients, including those whose beliefs diverge from those of the treating physician or from accepted medical advice.
- Remain sensitive to differences in patients' gender, age, race, culture, religion, and sexual orientation.
- Appreciate that informed adults with decision making capacity may refuse recommended medical treatment.
- Appreciate that physicians are not required to provide care that is medically futile.
- Demonstrate empathy for hospitalized patients.
- Endorse that physicians have an obligation not to discriminate against any patient or group of patients.

- Observe the boundaries of the physician-patient relationship.
- Promote cost effective care.
- Recognize the obligation to report fraud, professional misconduct, impairment, incompetence or abandonment of patients.
- Recognize potential conflicts of interest in accepting gifts and/or travel from commercial sources.
- Recognize potential individual and institutional conflicts of interest with incentive-based contractual agreements with pharmaceutical companies and other funding agents.
- Follow a systematic approach to risks, benefits and conflicts of interest in human subject research.
- Serve as a role model for professional and ethical conduct to house staff, medical students and other members of the interdisciplinary team.

QUALITY IMPROVEMENT

Quality improvement (QI) is the process of continually evaluating existing processes of care and developing new standards of practice. QI is influenced by objective data and focuses on systems change, rather than individual performance, in order to optimize performance and appropriate resource utilization. Hospitalists may lead or participate in QI teams to optimize management of common inpatient conditions and improve clinical outcomes based on standardized evidence based practices. Hospitalists should use evidence based outcomes data whenever available to support their inpatient practices and QI initiatives.

KNOWLEDGE

Hospitalists should be able to:
- Identify and categorize adverse outcomes that may include sentinel events, near misses, or other adverse events.
- Describe QI requirements for hospital accreditation that are supported by regulatory organizations.
- Describe outcome measurements currently studied by major payers and regulatory agencies.
- Identify guidelines and protocols supported by outcomes data to shape and standardize clinical practice.
- Describe and differentiate Root Cause Analysis (RCA) and Healthcare Failure Mode Effects Analysis (HFMEA) and their utility in quality improvement in the hospital setting.
- Describe the differences between outcome and process measures.
- List the characteristics of high-reliability organizations.
- Describe the elements of effective teams and teamwork.

SKILLS

Hospitalists should be able to:
- Apply current outcomes data and evidence based literature to individual hospitalist practice and systems improvements.
- Utilize quality data to define hospitalist practice.
- Express the relationship between value, quality and cost, and incorporate patient desires and satisfaction into the optimization of health care quality.
- Assess and incorporate new technology for systems improvement in hospital practice.
- Differentiate outcome measurements from process measurements.
- Interpret patient satisfaction metrics.

ATTITUDES

Hospitalists should be able to:
- Practice patient centered care and appreciate its value in improving patient safety and satisfaction.
- Apply the results of validated outcome studies to inpatient practice.
- Promote the adoption of new practices, guidelines and technology as supported by best available evidence.
- Structure QI initiatives that reflect evidence based literature and high quality outcomes data.
- Lead, coordinate or participate in the design and implementation of QI initiatives at individual, practice, and system levels, using a collaborative multidisciplinary team approach.
- Lead, coordinate or participate in Root Cause Analyses (RCA) and/or Healthcare Failure Mode Effects Analyses (HFMEA).
- Lead, coordinate or participate in outcomes monitoring at the institutional, regional and national levels, with an emphasis on development of standards and benchmarks.

RISK MANAGEMENT

Risk management seeks to reduce hazards to patients through a process identification, evaluation, and analysis of potential or actual adverse events. Hazard involves that harm that may occur as a result of healthcare delivery, which may be heightened in the hospital setting due to the higher acuity of patient illness, time pressures, and presence of trainees. Hospitalists should strive to comply with the letter and spirit of all applicable laws and regulations, avoid conflicts of interest, and conduct hospital business with integrity and ethical fervor. Hospitalists should also take a collaborative and proactive role with various services that may include risk management to help reduce risk in the hospital setting.

KNOWLEDGE

Hospitalists should be able to:
- Explain the legal definition of negligence and the concept of standard of care.
- Describe the effective components of informed consent.
- Explain the circumstances requiring informed consent.
- Describe HIPAA regulations related to patient confidentiality.
- Explain requirements for billing compliance.
- Describe other laws and regulations to the extent they are relevant to the practice of hospital medicine, including the Emergency Medical Treatment and Active Labor Act (EMTALA), the Patient Safety and Quality Improvement Act, and credentialing and licensing.
- Explain how ethical principles can be applied to risk management.

SKILLS

Hospitalists should be able to:
- Elicit informed consent from patients or surrogates for treatment plans and procedures when indicated.
- Provide adequate supervision of members of the patient care team, which may include physician assistants, fellows, residents or medical students.
- Apply guidelines of clinical ethics to patient care and risk management.
- Compare and minimize hazards of diagnostic and treatment management strategies for the individual patient.
- Ensure patient confidentiality.
- Comply with HIPAA regulations.
- Conduct medical practice and complete chart documentation to meet care needs and billing compliance, and reduce risks through effective communication.
- Conduct medical practice without violating any relevant laws or regulations.

ATTITUDES

Hospitalists should be able to:
- Apply ethical principles, which may include autonomy, beneficence, nonmaleficence, and justice, to promote patient centered care.
- Practice Hospital Medicine to meet or exceed accepted standards of care and reduce risk.
- Appreciate the importance of prompt, honest, and open discussions with patients and families regarding medical errors or harm.
- Respect patient wishes for treatment decisions and plans.
- Respect patient confidentiality.
- Collaborate with risk management in the required reporting and addressing of sentinel events or other medical errors.
- Lead, coordinate or participate in initiatives to improve and maintain HIPAA and billing compliance standards
- Lead, coordinate or participate in initiatives that result in processes of care that minimize risk.

TEAM APPROACH AND MULTIDSCIPLINARY CARE

Multidisciplinary care refers to active collaboration between various members in the healthcare system to develop optimal care plans for each hospitalized patient. Multidisciplinary care teams maintain goals to enhance quality and patient safety, improve outcomes, decrease length of stay, and lower costs. Hospitalists coordinate complex inpatient medical care from admission through all care transitions to discharge. Hospitalists lead multidisciplinary teams within their institutions to achieve these goals and to improve care processes.

KNOWLEDGE

Hospitalists should be able to:
- Describe the major elements of teamwork, including mutual respect, communication, common goals and plans, and accountability.
- List major barriers to effective team interactions.
- Describe aspects within an institution, including its local organizational culture, which can impact the structure and function of multidisciplinary teams.
- List factors that positively and negatively affect formation and effective performance of multidisciplinary teams.

SKILLS

Hospitalists should be able to:
- Determine an effective team composition and designate individual group member functions.
- Demonstrate group dynamic skills, including communication, negotiation, conflict resolution, delegation, and time management.
- Assess individual member's strengths and incorporate them effectively and productively into the team.
- Assess group dynamics and facilitate optimal team functioning.
- Integrate the assessments and recommendations of all contributing team members into the care plan.
- Conduct effective multidisciplinary team rounds, which may include patients and their families.
- Utilize team members' time effectively, maximizing efficiency and consistency.
- Ensure the delivery of timely and accurate information.
- Assess performance of team members, including self-assessment, and identify opportunities for improvement.

ATTITUDES

Hospitalists should be able to:
- Employ active listening techniques during interactions with team members and engage team participation.
- Communicate frequently with all members of the multidisciplinary team.
- Emphasize the importance of mutual respect among team members.
- Act as a role model in professional conflict resolution and discussion of disagreements.
- Share decision making responsibilities, within the appropriate scopes of practice, with care team members.
- Create an environment of shared responsibility with patients and caregivers, and provide opportunities for patient and/or caregivers to participate in medical decision making.
- Facilitate opportunities for interactive education among team members and for team members to educate patients and families.
- Coordinate seamless transitions of care by utilizing combined expertise of team members.
- Establish a hospital wide, non-punitive culture of error reporting and prevention.

TRANSITIONS OF CARE

The term "Transitions of Care" refers to specific interactions, communication, and planning required for patients to safely move from one service or setting to another. These transitions traditionally apply to transfers between the inpatient and outpatient setting. Transitions also occur between or within acute care facilities, and to or from subacute and non-acute facilities. Hospitalists provide leadership to promote efficient, safe transitions of care to ensure patient safety, reduce loss of information, and maintain the continuum of care.

KNOWLEDGE

Hospitalists should be able to:
- Define relevant information that should be retrieved and communicated during each care transition to ensure patient safety and maintain the continuum of care.
- Analyze potential strengths and limitations of patient transition processes.
- Describe the value of available ancillary services that can facilitate patient transitions.
- Distinguish available levels of care for patients and select the most appropriate option.
- Analyze strengths and limitations of different communication modalities utilized in patient transitions.

SKILLS

Hospitalists should be able to:
- Utilize the most efficient, effective, reliable and expeditious communication modalities for each care transition.
- Synthesize medical information received from referring physicians into care plan.
- Develop a care plan early during hospitalization that anticipates discharge or transfer needs.
- Organize and effectively communicate medical information in a succinct format for receiving clinicians.

ATTITUDES

Hospitalists should be able to:
- Appreciate the impact of care transitions on patient outcomes and satisfaction.
- Strive to utilize the best available communication modality in each care transition.
- Appreciate the value of *real time* interactive dialogue between clinicians during care transitions.
- Strive to personally communicate with every receiving or referring physician during care transitions.
- Appreciate the preferences of receiving physicians for transfer of information.
- Recognize the importance of a multidisciplinary approach to care transitions, including specifically nursing, rehabilitation, nutrition, pharmaceutical and social services.
- Expeditiously inform the primary care provider about significant changes in patient clinical status.
- Inform receiving physician of pending tests and determine who is responsible for checking results.
- Incorporate quality indicators for specific disease states and/or patient variables into discharge plans.
- Communicate with patients and families to explain their condition, ongoing medical regimens and therapies, follow-up care and available support services.
- Communicate with patients and families to explain clinical symptomatology that may require medical attention prior to scheduled follow-up.
- Anticipate and address language and/or literacy barriers to patient education.
- Prepare patients and families early in the hospitalization for anticipated care transitions.
- Review the discharge plans with patients, families, and healthcare team.
- Take responsibility to coordinate multidisciplinary teams early in the hospitalization course to facilitate patient education, optimize patient function, and improve discharge planning.
- Engage stakeholders in hospital initiatives to continuously assess the quality of care transitions.
- Lead, coordinate or participate in initiatives to develop and implement new protocols to improve or optimize transitions of care.
- Lead, coordinate or participate in evaluation of new strategies or information systems designed to improve care transitions.
- Maintain availability to discharged patients for questions during/between discharge and follow-up visit with receiving physician.

ABBREVIATIONS

ABG	Arterial blood gas
ACLS	Advanced cardiac life support
ACS	Acute coronary syndrome
ADE	Adverse drug event
ARF	Acute renal failures
ARR	Absolute risk reduction
BLS	Basic life support
CAD	Coronary artery disease
CAP	Community acquired pneumonia
CHF	Congestive heart failure
CNS	Central nervous system
COPD	Chronic obstructive pulmonary disease
CPOE	Computer physician order entry
CSF	Cerebrospinal fluid
CT	Computed tomography
CXR	Chest radiograph
DKA	Diabetic ketoacidosis
DSM-IV	Diagnostic and Statistical Manual of Mental Disorders (4th edition)
DVT	Deep vein thrombosis
EBM	Evidence based medicine
EKG	Electrocardiogram
FMEA	Failure mode and effects analysis
GI	Gastrointestinal
HAP	Hospital acquired pneumonia
HHS	Hyperglycemia hyperosmolar state
ICU	Intensive care unit
MRI	Magnetic resonance imaging
NNT	Number needed to treat
NSAIDs	Nonsteroidal anti-inflammatory drugs
NSTEMI	Non-ST-segment elevation myocardial infarction
OTC	Over-the-counter drugs
PBLI	Practice based learning and improvement
PE	Pulmonary embolus
PDI	Pneumonia severity index
PORT	Pneumonia patient outcomes research team
PDSA	Plan Do Study Act
PSI	Pneumonia Severity Index
QI	Quality Improvement
RCA	Root cause analysis
RRR	Relative risk reduction
RVU	Relative value units
STEMI	ST-elevation myocardial infarction
SIRS	Systemic Inflammatory Response Syndrome
UTI	Urinary tract infection
VTE	Venous thromboembolism

ORGANIZATIONS CITED IN TEXT

ABIM	American Board of Internal Medicine (www.abim.org)
ABP	American Board of Pediatrics (www.abp.org)
ACC	American College of Cardiology (www.acc.org)
ACGME	Accreditation Council for Graduate Medical Education (www.acgme.org)
ACLS	Advanced Cardiac Life Support (www.americanheart.org or www.acls.net)
ADA	American Diabetes Association (www.diabetes.org)
AHA	American Heart Association (www.americanheart.org)
AHRQ	Agency for Healthcare Research and Quality (www.ahrq.gov)
ATS	American Thoracic Society (www.thoracic.org)
BLS	Basic Life Support (www.americanheart.org or www.basiclifesupport.net)
CDCP	Centers for Disease Control and Prevention (www.cdc.gov)
EMTALA	Emergency Medical Treatment and Active Labor Act (www.emtala.com)
FDA	Food and Drug Administration (www.fda.gov)
HCUP	Healthcare Cost and Utilization Project (www.ahrq.gov/data/hcup)
HIPAA	Health Insurance Portability and Accountability Act (http://aspe.hhs.gov)
IASP	International Association for the Study of Pain (www.iasp-pain.org)
IDSA	Infectious Diseases Society of America (www.idsociety.org)
IOM	Institute of Medicine (www.iom.edu)
JCAHO	Joint Commission on Accreditation of Healthcare Organizations (www.jcaho.org)
NPSF	National Patient Safety Foundation (www.npsf.org)
NIS	Nationwide Inpatient Sample (www.hcup-us.ahrq.gov/nisoverview.jsp)
SHM	Society of Hospital Medicine (www.hospitalmedicine.org)
WHO	World Health Organization (www.who.int/en/)

Core Competencies in Hospital Medicine: Development and Methodology

Daniel D. Dressler, MD, MSc[1]
Michael J. Pistoria, DO, FACP[2]
Tina L. Budnitz, MPH[3]
Sylvia C. W. McKean, MD[4]
Alpesh N. Amin, MD, MBA, FACP [5]

[1] Department of Medicine, Emory University School of Medicine, Atlanta, Georgia

[2] Department of Medicine, Lehigh Valley Hospital, Allentown, Pennsylvania

[3] Society of Hospital Medicine, Philadelphia, Pennsylvania

[4] Department of Medicine, Harvard Medical School, Boston, Massachusetts

[5] Department of Medicine, University of California, Irvine, Orange, California

BACKGROUND: The hospitalist model of inpatient care has been rapidly expanding over the last decade, with significant growth related to the quality and efficiency of care provision. This growth and development have stimulated a need to better define and characterize the field of hospital medicine. Training and developing curricula specific to hospital medicine are the next step in the evolution of the field.

METHODS: *The Core Competencies in Hospital Medicine: A Framework for Curriculum Development* (the Core Competencies), by the Society of Hospital Medicine, introduces the expectations of hospitalists and provides an initial structural framework to guide medical educators in developing curricula that incorporate these competencies into the training and evaluation of students, clinicians-in-training, and practicing hospitalists. This article outlines the process that was undertaken to develop the Core Competencies, which included formation of a task force and editorial board, development of a topic list, the solicitation for and writing of chapters, and the execution of multiple reviews by the editorial board and both internal and external reviewers.

RESULTS: This process culminated in the Core Competencies document, which is divided into three sections: Clinical Conditions, Procedures, and Healthcare Systems. The chapters in each section delineate the core knowledge, skills, and attitudes necessary for effective inpatient practice while also incorporating a systems organization and improvement approach to care coordination and optimization.

CONCLUSIONS: These competencies should be a common reference and foundation for the creation of hospital medicine curricula and serve to standardize and improve inpatient training practices. *Journal of Hospital Medicine* 2006;1:48–56. © 2006 Society of Hospital Medicine.

KEYWORDS: medical education, curriculum.

Identification of the core competencies of a medical specialty provides the necessary framework for that specialty to develop, refine itself, and evolve. It also provides a structure from which training, testing, and curricula can be developed and effectively utilized. For nearly a decade, since the coining of the term *hospitalist*,[1] the field of hospital medicine has been emerging as the next generation of site-defined specialties, after emergency medicine and critical care medicine. *The Core Competencies in Hospital Medicine: A Framework for Curriculum Development* (referred to as the Core Competencies from this point on) introduces the expectations of hospitalists, helps to define their role, and suggests how knowledge, skill, and attitude acquisition might be evaluated. Furthermore, this document provides an initial structural framework from which curricula in adult hospital medicine may be developed.

This section is reprinted from the *Journal of Hospital Medicine,* Volume 1, Number 1, 2006, Pages 48–56. ©2006 Society of Hospital Medicine.

The Core Competencies document, produced by the Society of Hospital Medicine (SHM) and published as a supplement to the first issue of the *Journal of Hospital Medicine*,[2] is meant to serve as a framework for educators at all levels of medical education to develop curricula, training, and evaluations for students, clinicians-in-training, and practicing hospitalists. The Core Competencies document is not meant to contain a complete compilation of inpatient clinical topics or to re-create what many residency training programs in adult inpatient care already provide. It should not limit and does not define every aspect of hospitalist practice. It includes the most common and fundamental elements of inpatient care without exhaustively listing every clinical entity that may be encountered by a hospitalist. Some of the more common clinical topics encountered by inpatient physicians are included, with an emphasis on subject areas that stress a systems-based approach to health care, which is central to the practice of hospital medicine. This initial version of the Core Competencies document also focuses on potential areas of deficiency in the training of physicians to become hospitalists. It provides developers of curricula and content with a standardized set of measurable learning objectives, while allowing them the flexibility needed to address specific contexts and incorporate advances in medicine.

The SHM, the sole professional organization representing inpatient physicians, defines hospitalists as "physicians whose primary professional focus is the general medical care of hospitalized patients. Their activities include patient care, teaching, research, and leadership related to Hospital Medicine."[3] An estimated 12,000 hospitalists are currently practicing in the United States, with a projected workforce need of an estimated 20,000–30,000 practicing hospitalists in the United States in the next 5–10 years.[4] Various factors have contributed to the rapid growth and expansion of hospital medicine, including factors related to care efficiency, care quality, and inpatient teaching.[5–12] The pressures that have contributed to the development of and evolution toward the hospitalist model of care over the past decade are facilitating the transformation from a traditional model of inpatient care to the care of inpatients by hospitalist physicians dedicated primarily to the inpatient setting. As a result of this growth in hospital medicine, the SHM realized that core competencies were needed to help define the field.

The purpose of this article is to describe the developmental process and content structure of the Core Competencies document. It delineates the process from initial needs assessment to topic list development to chapter production to internal and external review and revisions of individual chapters and the complete document. The supplement to this first issue of the *Journal of Hospital Medicine* contains 1) the Core Competencies,[2] 2) a reprint of this article, and 3) a reprint of the article by McKean et al. in this issue detailing how to use the Core Competencies,[13] with examples and suggestions related to curriculum development. The authors propose that this combined compilation may spur curriculum development in hospital medicine that will help to define the field and set expectations for practice.

PROCESS AND TIMELINE
Education Summit
Early in the growth of hospital medicine, the Society of Hospital Medicine identified a need to better define a common educational and practice framework for hospitalist physicians. Such a framework could help to define hospitalists as a distinct group of practicing physicians with common goals and a common set of competencies. The importance of identifying and delineating the common knowledge, skills, and attitudes of hospitalists was paramount. Figure 1 shows the details of the 4-year process of developing the Core Competencies.

In 2002, the SHM drew together educational leaders in hospital medicine in its first educational summit. One of the primary charges that the SHM received from this summit was to develop the needed core curriculum in hospital medicine. After the summit, the SHM's Education Committee formed the Core Curriculum Task Force (CCTF), composed of approximately 15 member hospitalists, with representation from university and community hospitals, teaching and nonteaching programs, and for-profit and not-for-profit settings from various geographic regions of the country. The selection process ensured that the task force was representative of practicing hospitalists and SHM membership throughout the United States.

The CCTF
The task force met through frequent conference-call meetings and at least one in-person meeting annually. The primary goal set forth by the task force was the initial development of a distinct set of

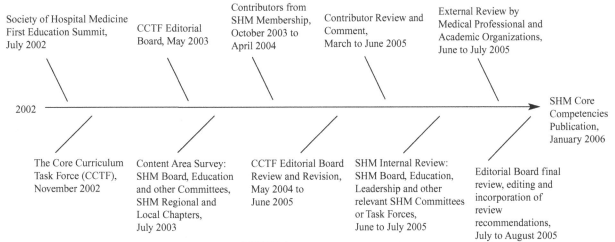

FIGURE 1. Process and timeline.

core competencies in hospital medicine that could then guide curriculum development within the field.

Topic List

The task force determined that the topics (or chapters) should be divided into three sections—Clinical Conditions, Procedures, and Healthcare Systems (Table 1, Chapter List)—all integral components of the practice of hospital medicine. For Clinical Conditions chapters, the task force decided that an exhaustive listing of all potential clinical entities that hospitalists might encounter during their clinical practice was not the goal of the Core Competencies. Rather, clinical topics were selected to reflect conditions in the hospital setting that are encountered with significant frequency, that might be significantly life-threatening, or that are likely to have the significant involvement and impact of hospitalists in altering or refining care processes, leading to improvement in care quality and efficiency. The list of Clinical Condition chapters should not limit or rigidly define the scope of practice of hospitalist physicians. Instead, it should help those entering the field of hospital medicine better understand some of the core clinical topics on which hospitalists focus in the design of institutional or global quality initiatives.

Clinical Conditions Section

In an effort to both narrow and delineate the core Clinical Condition areas necessary for practicing hospital medicine, the task force elected first to draw from national data the most common diagnosis-related groups (DRGs) discharged from U.S. hospitals. Utilizing the Medicare database, the top 15 nonsurgical discharge diagnoses were initially selected. Certain clinical conditions that the task force believed to be highly relevant to the practice of hospital medicine but that did not neatly fall into a specific DRG, such as pain management and perioperative medicine, were proposed for and then added to the list of Clinical Conditions chapters by the task force. Other chapters, such as that on venous thromboembolism, were added because a particular disease, although not necessarily a high-ranked discharge DRG, showed high inpatient morbidity and mortality and reflected the role of the hospitalist in the prevention of predictable complications during hospitalization. When possible, some diagnoses were consolidated to better incorporate crosscutting competencies or to highlight opportunities for leadership in systems-based improvements. For example, upper and lower gastrointestinal bleeding were consolidated into the chapter on gastrointestinal bleeding. Similarly, all relevant arrhythmias that a hospitalist might encounter were consolidated into a single chapter. For at least one clinical topic, pneumonia, the task force believed it necessary to have two distinct chapters, one on community-acquired pneumonia and the other on hospital-acquired pneumonia, because these two entities are significantly different and have distinct competencies. The final listing of Clinical Conditions chapters reflects 19 clinical areas that hospitalists encounter on a frequent basis

TABLE 1
List of Chapters of the Core Competencies in Hospital Medicine

Clinical Conditions*	Procedures	Healthcare Systems
Acute Coronary Syndrome	Arthrocentesis	Care of the Elderly Patient
Acute Renal Failure	Chest Radiograph Interpretation	Care of Vulnerable Populations
Alcohol and Drug Withdrawal	Electrocardiogram Interpretation	Communication
Asthma	Emergency Procedures	Diagnostic Decision Making
Cardiac Arrhythmia	Lumbar Puncture	Drug Safety, Pharmacoeconomics and Pharmacoepidemiology
Cellulitis	Paracentesis	Equitable Allocation of Resources
Chronic Obstructive Pulmonary Disease	Thoracentesis	Evidence-Based Medicine
Community-Acquired Pneumonia	Vascular Access	Hospitalist as Consultant
Congestive Heart Failure		Hospitalist as Teacher
Delirium and Dementia		Information Management
Diabetes Mellitus		Leadership
Gastrointestinal Bleed		Management Practices
Hospital-Acquired Pneumonia		Nutrition and the Hospitalized Patient
Pain Management		Palliative Care
Perioperative Medicine		Patient Education
Sepsis Syndrome		Patient Handoff
Stroke		Patient Safety
Urinary Tract Infection		Practice-Based Learning and Improvement
Venous Thromboembolism		Prevention of Healthcare–Associated Infections and Antimicrobial Resistance
		Professionalism and Medical Ethics
		Quality Improvement
		Risk Management
		Team Approach and Multidisciplinary Care
		Transitions of Care

*Clinical chapter list is not a complete compilation of all inpatient clinical conditions that hospitalists may find in an inpatient setting.

and for which they can have an effect on systems and processes of care. These clinical chapters form a foundation of topics for which hospitalists have already begun quality and efficiency initiatives.

The task force further decided that symptom evaluation and management could be consolidated into a systems chapter dedicated to diagnostic decision making. A reasonably large constellation of symptoms, including but not limited to chest pain, shortness of breath, syncope, and altered mental status, are encountered by hospitalists daily. Although evaluation and management of these symptoms are extremely important parts of triage, subsequent testing, and hospital care, the ability to develop a differential diagnosis and proceed with the indicated testing and its interpretation is common to all symptom evaluation. Such evaluation and diagnostic decision making are therefore summarized in a single chapter in the Healthcare Systems section, and no symptom chapters are found in the Clinical section.

Procedures Section
The initial topic lists for the Procedures and Systems sections were developed through input from the broad representation of the Core Curriculum Task Force. The chapters in the Procedures section contain competencies expected for the inpatient procedures that hospitalists are most likely to perform or supervise in their day-to-day care of hospitalized patients. The presence of a procedural skill in the Core Competencies does not necessarily indicate that every hospitalist will perform or be proficient in that procedure. Similarly, the absence of a procedure from the Core Competencies should not exclude trained and experienced hospitalists from performing that procedure. The task force recognizes that the individual hospital setting, including local and regional variations, determines who might perform certain procedures depending on many factors, which may include whether there are trainees, specialty support including radiology, and procedure teams. The Procedures section outlines those procedures frequently performed in the everyday practice of hospital medicine and incorporates relevant competencies to afford proper performance, patient education and in-

volvement, prevention of complications, and quality improvement for these procedures.

Healthcare Systems Section

Although many competencies delineated in the Clinical Conditions and Procedures sections of the supplement may be taught well during medical school and residency training, that is not true of the chapters and competencies in the Healthcare Systems section, many of which are not extensively taught in most undergraduate or graduate medical education programs. Therefore, many hospitalists must gain or supplant their knowledge, skills, and attitudes in system areas posttraining.

The Healthcare Systems section delineates themes integral to the successful practice of hospital medicine in diverse hospital settings. Many chapters in this section focus on processes and systems of care that typically span multiple disease entities and frequently require multidisciplinary input to create a coordinated effort for care quality and efficiency. The chapters and core competencies in the Healthcare Systems section direct hospitalists to lead and innovate in their own hospital practices and to convey the principles of evidence-based inpatient medical care and systems-based practice to medical students, physicians-in-training, other medical staff, colleagues, and patients. The task force expects that many new hospitalists will still be learning many of the competencies in the Healthcare Systems section during the early stages of their posttraining practice. However, as training of hospitalists during undergraduate and graduate medical education further evolves, we expect that more hospitalists will enter the workforce with more of the skills necessary to prepare them for their careers.

Some Healthcare Systems chapters have clinical themes but were included in this section because it is believed that the clinical approach always spans multiple clinical entities and always requires an organizational approach crossing several disciplines in medicine in order to optimize the hospital care. Such chapters include Care of the Elderly Patient, Prevention of Healthcare Associated Infections and Antimicrobial Resistance, Nutrition and the Hospitalized Patient, and Palliative Care. Other chapters in the Healthcare Systems section focus on educational themes that drive the practice of hospital medicine and the lifelong learning and teaching required of hospitalists. Some of these chapters include Evidence-Based Medicine,

Hospitalist as Teacher, Patient Education, and Practice-Based Learning and Improvement. Still other chapters in the Healthcare Systems section identify much of the organizational approach—both from clinical practice and practice management standpoints—that must be adopted by hospitalists in order to provide high-quality care while maintaining functional and sound practice. Examples of chapters focusing on clinical practice organization include Patient Safety, Quality Improvement, Team Approach and Multidisciplinary Care, Transitions of Care, and Patient Handoffs. Although the Transitions of Care chapter focuses on the processes and communication required for the safe transition of patients from one clinical setting to another; the Patient Handoffs (or "sign-out") chapter focuses on the hospitalist-to-hospitalist communication essential when one hospitalist assumes care of a patient from another (either from dayshift to nightshift on the same service or assuming care of service from a different service). Examples of chapters focusing on practice management organization include Business Practices, Equitable Allocation of Resources, Leadership, and Risk Management. Overall, the Healthcare Systems chapters help to characterize and delineate the practice and scope of hospital medicine, especially with topics not taught in detail during most residency training programs.

Editorial Board, Content Survey, and Topic List Refinement

Once the initial topic list was created, a five-member editorial board was chosen from the CCTF membership, including the SHM CCTF chair, the Education Committee chair, two member hospitalists, and a health education specialist. The purpose of this board was to interpret survey feedback, solicit contributors to write competency chapters, review and revise the chapters submitted, and prepare the larger document for review and final publication. The Core Curriculum Task Force developed a survey to obtain feedback on the initial topic list. Face validity was established through a survey sent electronically in 2003 to the SHM Board of Directors and Education Committee, as well as to 10 representatives of each SHM regional council and local chapter. In all, more than 250 hospitalists representing diverse geographic and practice backgrounds were surveyed. Feedback from the survey was reviewed by the CCTF. The topic list was then revised with additions and modifications incorporated from survey feedback. The scope of individual topics also was modified in multiple iterations congruent with the internal and external review processes.

Contributors

Contributors were solicited by the task force, utilizing SHM databases—believed to be the most comprehensive registry of hospitalist physicians—and an electronic call for nominations to practicing hospitalists from around the United States. Other recognized content experts were solicited independently on the basis of chapter or content needs. Efforts were taken to identify hospitalists with expertise in specific topic areas, particularly those with a history of presentations or publications on individual chapter subject matter. Potential contributors submitted credentials, including curricula vitae and other supporting documents or information, when requesting to write a specific chapter for the Core Competencies compendium. Contributors were competitively selected on the basis of their submitted information compared to those of others requesting to write the same chapter. In some cases practicing hospitalists were paired with nonhospitalist expert contributors to create a chapter. Contributors were provided with guidelines with which to prepare their chapter.

Review and Revision

The editorial board reviewed all the chapters, rigorously evaluating each chapter through at least five stages of review and revision. First, chapters were reviewed by the editorial board—initially by at least two physician members and then by the entire editorial board. Chapters were reviewed for the scope and completeness of concepts, adherence to educational theory, and consistency in chapter format. Changes in content and for consistency were extensive in some chapters, whereas others required only small or moderate changes. Significant editing was required to create chapters as a compilation of specific, measurable competencies as opposed to topic-related content. All chapters required some level of modification to assist with consistency in style, language, and overall goals. Where appropriate, individual chapters were also reviewed by relevant SHM committees, task forces, or content experts, and initial feedback was provided. For example, the Leadership chapter was reviewed by the SHM Leadership Task Force. Other SHM committees and task forces involved in chap-

ter reviews included the Education, Healthcare Quality and Patient Safety, and Ethics committees as well as the Geriatric Task Force. Changes recommended changes on the basis of committee and task force feedback were incorporated into the relevant chapters.

Second, revisions of individual chapters from the editorial board were sent back to contributors for final comment, revision, and approval. Third, the compilation of all chapters and sections was reviewed (as a whole) and underwent further revision by the editorial board based on feedback from the contributors and the relevant SHM committees. Fourth, the entire revised supplement was sent for an internal review by the SHM board and relevant SHM committees or committee representatives.

Fifth, final reviews were solicited from external reviewers of medical professional organizations and academic organizations. Feedback from the internal and external reviews were compiled and systematically evaluated by the CCTF editorial board. Recommended changes were incorporated into individual chapters or throughout the Core Competencies compendium on the basis of the evaluation and consensus approval of the editorial board. For example, one reviewer believed that quality improvement initiatives were necessary for all procedures that hospitalists perform in order to help reduce the risk of complications. Therefore, each procedure chapter was revised to reflect this competency. Similarly, another reviewer thought that in many chapters the involvement of nursing and other medical staff in the implementation of multidisciplinary teams was underemphasized. Therefore, efforts were taken to improve the emphasis of these key participants in multidisciplinary hospital care.

The efforts of many individuals and professional organizations have helped the CCTF to refine the expectations of a professional trained in the discipline of hospital medicine. Table 2 has a complete listing of those solicited to be internal and external reviewers. Although aggressive efforts were undertaken to encourage feedback from all solicited reviewers of the Core Competencies document, time or other constraints prevented some reviewers from responding to the review request (overall response or review rate: 52%). Nevertheless, the multiple review and revision process brought what was initially disparate content and organization together in a much more cohesive and consistent

- Accreditation Council of Graduate Medical Education (ACGME)
- Agency for Healthcare Research & Quality (AHRQ)
- American Academy of Family Practice (AAFP)
- American Association of Critical Care Nurses (AACCN)
- American Association of Subspecialty Professors
- American Board of Family Practice
- American Board of Internal Medicine (ABIM)
- American College of Chest Physicians (ACCP)
- American College of Emergency Physicians (ACEP)
- American College of Physicians (ACP)
- American Geriatrics Society
- American Hospital Association (AHA)
- Association of American Medical Colleges (AAMC)
- Institute for Healthcare Improvement (IHI)
- John A. Hartford Foundation
- Joint Commission on Accreditation of Healthcare Organizations (JCAHO)
- Residency Review Committee – Internal Medicine (RRC-IM)
- Reynolds Foundation
- Robert Wood Johnson Foundation (RWJF)
- Society of Critical Care Medicine (SCCM)
- Society of General Internal Medicine (SGIM)
- Society of Hospital Medicine
- ○ Board of Directors (9 members solicited)
- ○ CCTF Members (3 members solicited exclusive of editorial board)

*Response rate: 52%

approach and structure to competencies in hospital medicine.

CHAPTER CONTENT DESCRIPTION

As previously delineated, the Core Competencies document has three sections: Clinical Conditions, Procedures, and Healthcare Systems. The chapters in the entire compendium and within each section have been designed to stand alone and to be used either individually or collectively to assist with curriculum development in hospital medicine. However, each chapter should be used in the context of the entire document because a particular issue may only be touched on in one chapter but may be more elaborately detailed in another. For example, all clinical conditions chapters include a competency on the issue of care transitions, but the specific competencies for care transitions are presented in a separate Transitions of Care chapter.

All chapters in each section begin with an introduction that provides brief background information and establishes the relevance of the topic to practicing hospitalists. Each chapter then utilizes the educational theory of learning domains. The learning domains include the cognitive domain (knowledge), the psychomotor domain (skills), and the affective domain (attitudes). The companion article "How to Use *The Core Competencies in Hospital Medicine: A Framework for Curriculum Development*"[13] describes in detail the educational theory guiding the development of the Core Competencies document and suggested methods for applying it to the development and revision of curricula and other training activities.

The task force further decided that each chapter in the Clinical Conditions and Procedures sections should include a subsection dedicated to system organization and improvement, an added domain that requires integration of knowledge, skills, and attitudes and the involvement of other medical services and disciplines for optimal patient care. The editorial board believed that system organization and improvement was already an intrinsic feature embedded in the chapters of the Healthcare Systems section. Therefore, this subsection was not included in those chapters.

Hospitalists subscribe to a systems organizational approach to clinical management and processes of care within the hospital. This systems approach, more than any level of knowledge or skill, is required to effectively and efficiently practice in the hospital setting. Practicing with a systems approach, with the interest of improving processes of care, is embedded throughout the Core Competencies document and is a practice method that all hospitalists may strive to achieve as they develop and improve their inpatient care. The competencies within the Systems Organization and Improvement section may contain a range of competency expectation (eg, lead, coordinate, *or* participate in...) to acknowledge their uniqueness and variation according to practice settings and locally instituted responsibilities.

Each competency within a chapter details a level of proficiency, providing guidance on learning activities and potential evaluation strategies. Several overarching themes are followed in the chapters that help to define hospitalists as physicians who specialize in the care of hospitalized patients. First, hospitalists strive to support and adhere to a multidisciplinary approach for the patients under their care. Such an approach involves active interaction with and integration of other hospital medical staff (eg, nursing, rehabilitation therapies, social services) and of specialty medical or surgical services when indicated. Recognizing that hospitalists vary in experience and mastery of their field, the task force and editorial board believed that, at minimum, hospitalists would participate in multidisciplinary teams for improvement of the care and process related to the clinical conditions within their organization. However, they might also lead and/or coordinate teams in such efforts. Therefore, most chapters contain competencies that expect hospitalists to "lead, coordinate, or participate..." in multidisciplinary teams or initiatives that will facilitate optimal care within their organization.

Second, because hospital medicine centers around the quality of inpatient care, participation in quality improvement (QI) initiatives, focusing on improving processes or systems of care in a local institution or organization, may be common in hospitalist practices. The level of involvement and role in QI initiatives may vary according to the particular system, the resources available, and a hospitalist's experience. Finally, because hospitalist care intrinsically involves an increase in the number of care transitions and handoffs, hospitalists need to remain sensitive to and focused on the care transitions that occur with their patients. Such transitions may occur as patients enter the hospital, move from one location to another within the hospital, or leave the hospital. This vulnerable time for patients requires hospitalists to be vigilant in their communication efforts—with patients, with medical staff, and with outpatient clinicians.

Each competency was crafted to indicate the relevant concept, the level of proficiency expected, and a way to evaluate mastery. The teaching processes and learning experiences that must take place to achieve competency are left for curriculum developers and instructors to design. These core competencies represent an initial step in curriculum development, creating an identity and core set of expectations for hospitalists that we believe will lead to progress and maturity within the field.

SUMMARY AND FUTURE DIRECTIONS
The practice of hospital medicine requires proficiency of interrelated aspects of practice—clinical, procedural, and system-based competencies. For practicing hospitalists, the Core Competencies document may serve as a resource to refine skills and assist in program development at individual institutions, both regionally and nationally. For residency program directors and clerkship directors, the Core Competencies document can function as a

guide for developing the curriculum of inpatient medicine rotations or for meeting the requirements of the Outcomes Project of the Accreditation Council on Graduate Medical Education's. Last, for those developing continuing medical education programs, the Core Competencies document or individual chapters or topics within it may serve as an outline around which specific or broad-based programs can be developed. Although the development of such curricula and the recipients of them should be evaluated, the actual evaluation is left to the curriculum developers.

Hospitalists are invested in making hospitals run better. They are positioned to take leadership roles in addressing quality, efficiency, and cost interests in both community and academic hospital settings. Their goals include improving care processes, hospital work life, and the setting in which they practice. The key core competencies described in this compendium define hospitalists as agents of change 1) to develop and implement systems to enable best practices to occur from admission through discharge, and 2) to promote the development of a safer culture within the hospital.

Hospital medicine remains an evolving specialty. Although great care was taken to construct these competencies so they would retain their relevance over time, SHM, the Core Curriculum Task Force, and the editorial board recognize the need for their continual reevaluation and modification in the context of advances and changes in the practice of hospital medicine. Our intent is that these competencies be a common reference and foundation for the creation of hospital medicine curricula and serve to standardize and improve training practices.

Address for correspondence and reprint requests: Daniel D. Dressler, MD, MSc, Hospital Medicine Service, Emory University Hospital, Emory University School of Medicine, 1364 Clifton Rd., P.O. Box M7, Atlanta, GA 30322; Fax: (404) 712-1804; E-mail: Daniel.Dressler@Emoryhealthcare.org

Received 27 August 2005; revision received 21 October 2005; accepted 6 November 2005.

REFERENCES
1. Wachter RM, Goldman L. The emerging role of "hospitalists" in the American health care system. *N Engl J Med.* 1996;335:514–517.
2. Pistoria MJ, Amin AN, Dressler DD, McKean SCW, Budnitz TL, eds. *The Core Competencies in Hospital Medicine: A Framework for Curriculum Development. J Hosp Med.* 2006; 1(supplement 1).
3. Society of Hospital Medicine. About SHM: What is a hospitalist? Available from URL: http://www.hospitalmedicine.org [accessed July 22, 2005].

4. Williams MV. The future of hospital medicine: evolution or revolution? *Am J Med.* 2004;117:446–450.
5. Wachter RM, Goldman L. The hospitalist movement 5 years later. *JAMA.* 2002;287:487–494.
6. Auerbach AD, Wachter RM, Katz P, et al. Implementation of a voluntary hospitalist service at a community teaching hospital: improved clinical efficiency and patient outcomes. *Ann Intern Med.* 2002;137:859–865.
7. Meltzer D, Manning WG, Morrison J, et al. Effects of physician experience on costs and outcomes on an academic general medicine service: results of a trial of hospitalists. *Ann Intern Med.* 2002;137:866–874.
8. Shojania KG, Duncan BW, McDonald KM, et al. Making Healthcare aafer: a critical analysis of patient safety practices. Rockville, MD: U.S. Dept. of Health and Human Services, Agency for Healthcare Research and Quality; 2001. AHRQ publication 01-E058. Available from URL: http://www.ahrq.gov.
9. Hunter AJ, Desai SS, Harrison RA, et al. Medical student evaluation of the quality of hospitalist and nonhospitalist teaching faculty on inpatient medicine rotations. *Acad Med.* 2004;79:78–82.
10. Kripalani S, Pope AC, Rask K, et al. Hospitalists as teachers. *J Gen Intern Med.* 2004;19(1):8–15.
12. Kulaga ME, Charney P, O'Mahony SP, et al. The positive impact of initiation of hospitalist clinician educators. *J Gen Intern Med.* 2004;19:293–301.
12. Hauer KE, Wachter RM, McCulloch CE, et al. Effects of hospitalist attending physicians on trainee satisfaction with teaching and with internal medicine rotations. *Arch Intern Med.* 2004;164:1866–1887.
13. McKean SCW, Budnitz TL, Dressler DD, Amin AN, Pistoria MJ. How to use *The Core Competencies in Hospital Medicine: A Framework for Curriculum Development. J Hosp Med.* 2006;1:57–67.

How to Use *The Core Competencies in Hospital Medicine: A Framework for Curriculum Development*

Sylvia C. W. McKean, MD[1]
Tina L. Budnitz, MPH[2]
Daniel D. Dressler, MD, MSc[3]
Alpesh N. Amin, MD, MBA, FACP[4]
Michael J. Pistoria, DO, FACP[5]

[1] Department of Medicine, Harvard Medical School, Boston, Massachusetts

[2] Society of Hospital Medicine, Philadelphia, Pennsylvania

[3] Department of Medicine, Emory University School of Medicine, Atlanta, Georgia

[4] Department of Medicine, University of California, Irvine, Orange, California

[5] Department of Medicine, Lehigh Valley Hospital, Allentown, Pennsylvania

BACKGROUND: The seminal article that coined the term *hospitalist,* published in 1996, attributed the role of the hospitalist to enhancing throughput and cost reduction, primarily through reduction in length of stay, accomplished by having a dedicated clinician on site in the hospital. Since that time the role of the hospitalist has evolved, and hospitalists are being called upon to demonstrate that they actually improve quality of care and the education of the next generation of physicians. A companion article in this issue describes in detail the rationale for the development of the Core Competencies document and the methods by which it was created.

METHODS: Specific cases that hospitalists may encounter in their daily practice are used to illustrate how the Core Competencies can be applied to curriculum development. The cases illustrate 1) a specific problem and the need for improvement; 2) a needs assessment of the targeted learners (hospitalists and clinicians in training); 3) goals and specific measurable objectives; 4) educational strategies using the competencies to provide structure and guidance; 5) implementation (applying competencies to a variety of training opportunities and curricula); 6) evaluation and feedback; and 7) remaining questions and the need for additional research.

RESULTS: This article illustrates how to utilize *The Core Competencies in Hospital Medicine* to educate trainees and faculty, to prioritize educational scholarship and research strategies, and thus to improve the care of our patients.

CONCLUSIONS: Medical educators should compare their learning objectives to the Core Competencies to ensure that their trainees have achieved competency to practice hospital medicine and improve the hospital setting. *Journal of Hospital Medicine* 2006;1:57–67. © *2006 Society of Hospital Medicine.*

KEYWORDS: core competencies, curricula development, education, hospital medicine.

T he seminal article that coined the term *hospitalist,* in 1996, attributed the role of the hospitalist to enhancing throughput and cost reduction, primarily through reduction in length of stay, accomplished by having a dedicated clinician on site in the hospital.[1] Since that time the role of the hospitalist has evolved to address the needs of multiple stakeholders at a time when traditional residency programs in inpatient adult medicine do not adequately train physicians to become effective agents of change in complex and potentially unsafe hospital systems. Continuing the trend of pediatrics, obstetrics, gynecology, and geriatrics, hospitalists have emerged as a distinct group of physicians who fill a needed clinical niche and are demonstrating the benefits of bringing a unique role and skill sets to the general hospital ward.[2]

The eligibility requirements for certification by the American

This section is reprinted from the *Journal of Hospital Medicine,* Volume 1, Number 1, 2006, Pages 57–67. ©2006 Society of Hospital Medicine.

Board of Internal Medicine specify that the discipline "must 1) have a distinct and unique body of knowledge, 2) have clinical applicability sufficient to support a distinct clinical practice, 3) generate new information and research, 4) require a minimum training period of 12 months, and 5) have a substantial number of trainees and training programs nationwide."[3] The Society of Hospital Medicine (SHM), the national professional organization of hospitalists, commissioned a task force to develop *The Core Competencies in Hospital Medicine: A Framework for Curriculum Development* (referred to from here on as the Core Competencies) to standardize the expectations of practicing hospitalists, serve as a foundation for curricula and other professional development experiences, prioritize educational scholarship and research strategies, and assess the adequacy and improvement opportunities for current training and accreditation of hospital medicine physicians.[4] The preceding companion article "The Core Competencies in Hospital Medicine: Development and Methodology," describes in detail the rationale for the development of the Core Competencies and the methods by which the document was created.[5]

PURPOSE

The purpose of this article is to illustrate how curriculum developers can apply the *Core Competencies in Hospital Medicine* to educate trainees and faculty, to prioritize educational scholarship and research strategies, and thus to improve the care of our patients.

TARGET AUDIENCE

The Core Competencies specifically targets directors of continuing medical education (CME), hospitalist programs and fellowships, residency programs, and medical school internal medicine clerkships. It is also intended for health educators, hospital administrators, potential employers, policy makers, and agencies funding quality-improvement initiatives in the hospital setting. For residency program directors and clerkship directors, the chapters can guide in the development of curricula for inpatient medicine rotations or in meeting the Accreditation Council on Graduate Medical Education's Outcomes Project. For directors developing medical education curricula, *The Core Competencies in Hospital Medicine* can serve as a template for CME. For hospitalists, hospital administrators, and potential employers, the Core Competencies can be used to as the starting point in local

program development and as a resource for refining the skills of all hospitalists, even very experienced practicing clinicians.

DEFINITION OF CORE COMPETENCIES IN HOSPITAL MEDICINE

The Core Competencies in Hospital Medicine provides a framework for curricular development based on a shared understanding of the essential knowledge, skills, and attitudes expected of physicians working as hospitalists. The development process will be ongoing, with revisions reflecting the evolving specialty of hospital medicine, the needs of practicing hospitalists, and feedback from users of the Core Competencies.

PROBLEM IDENTIFICATION AND GENERAL NEEDS ASSESSMENT

Delivery of health care has large gaps compared to ideal performance. Since the publication by the Institute of Medicine of *To Err Is Human*, in 1999, multiple agencies including the American Hospital Association, the National Quality Forum, and the U.S. Agency for Health Care Research and Quality (AHRQ) have reported on the incidence of medical errors in U.S. hospitals.[6,7] Recognizing that medical errors represent a major health concern in the United States, the Joint Commission on the Accreditation of Health Care Organizations (JCAHO) now requires patient safety initiatives for hospital accreditation.[8] Problem-based learning and improvement and systems based practice are now required competencies in medical residency curricula by the Accreditation Council for Graduate Medical Education (ACGME) and these requirements have led to the development of continuous quality techniques for preventing errors and a variety of patient safety initiatives.[9]

In 2002 the SHM recognized the need for identifying a distinct set of competencies in hospital medicine. The published competencies highlight the current gap in training of hospitalists and the imperative for revising curricula relating to inpatient care, hospital systems, and teaching.[4] With adequate training and preparation, hospitalists can take the lead in implementing systems for best practices from admission through discharge and care transition, and they can direct the development of a safer, more patient-centered, and cost-efficient culture.

By defining the role of the hospitalist, the Core Competencies reflects the view of the SHM about what is possible but does not suggest how a training program might be modified to achieve desired outcomes or provide any content, resources, or teaching strategies. It will be up to curriculum developers to determine the scope of cognitive, psychomotor, and affective objectives that targeted learners—hospitalists, residents, and other members of the multidisciplinary team—should be required to acquire through lectures, discussions, syllabus material, clinical experience, and other venues. We agree with a broader definition of the term *curriculum* for graduate medical education, one that "goes beyond curriculum as a plan and takes into account the learners' experiences, both planned and unplanned" in the hospital setting.[10] "In contrast to the technologic theory of curriculum, in which lists of knowledge and skills represent final destinations, in the experiential model of curriculum, the lists provide only points of departure."[11] The goal of the Core Competencies is to facilitate curriculum development using complex teaching environments as building blocks through which learning can occur.

CORE COMPETENCIES FOR HOSPITALISTS: OVERVIEW

The Core Competencies in Hospital Medicine is the first published competency-based framework for professional development of hospitalists and provides the basis for accreditation in hospital medicine.[12] The Core Competencies is organized into three sections—Clinical Conditions, Procedures, and Healthcare Systems. The supplement intentionally does not focus on content; rather, specific competencies describe unambiguous, measurable learning objectives. Each chapter can be used as a stand-alone chapter to develop training and curricula for a particular topic area. Each chapter divides competencies into three domains of educational outcomes: cognitive (knowledge), affective (attitudes), and psychomotor (skills). Each domain has defined levels of proficiency going from knowledge, the lowest level, to evaluation, the highest.[12,13] A specific level of proficiency is articulated in the competencies through careful selection of corresponding action verbs, which clearly indicate how mastery could be assessed (see Table 1).

In addition to specific competencies in these commonly accepted learning domains, the Clinical Conditions and Procedure sections of the Core Competencies articulate the proficiencies that hospitalists should possess in systems organization and improvement. The clinical topics were selected to set expectations of leading or participating in system improvements specific to a clinical area and

TABLE 1
Establishing Proficiency within a Competency

GI Bleed Example—Levels of Proficiency in the Cognitive Domain (Knowledge)	
UNDERSTAND the advantages and disadvantages of medical, endoscopic, and surgical treatments for patients with upper and lower GI bleeding	The first option, use of the verb *understand* gives little insight into level of proficiency. A patient could read a list on a pamphlet and truthfully claim to have achieved "understanding" of the advantages of each approach. An experienced gastroenterologist could make the same claim. Yet the two obviously differ in their level of comprehension.
LIST the advantages and disadvantages of medical, endoscopic, and surgical treatments for patients with upper and lower GI bleeding	In the second option, use of the verb *list* indicates that the expectation for a learner is to be able to literally make a quick list of advantages, perhaps merely regurgitating what was read in a text, indicating the lowest level of learning outcome, or *knowledge*.
COMPARE the advantages and disadvantages of medical, endoscopic, and surgical treatments for patients with upper and lower GI bleeding	In this option, use of the verb *compare* indicates that a clinician must be able to grasp the meaning of material and consider all options, indicating a higher level of learning outcome, or *comprehension*.

Although the differences in these statements may seem subtle, they are essential to discerning a level of proficiency. Verbs that convey higher levels of proficiency in the cognitive domain include:
- *Apply*, or the ability to use learned material in new and concrete situations,
- *Analyze*, which requires an understanding of both content and its organizational structure,
- *Synthesize*, or the ability to create new patterns of structures, and
- *Evaluate*, or the ability to judge the value of material (statement, research) for a given purpose, the highest level.

Learning outcomes in the evaluation category are the highest because they contain elements of all other categories plus conscious value judgments based on clearly defined criteria.[13]

Each competency in the Core Competencies was crafted to indicate the relevant concept, its level of proficiency, and how mastery could be evaluated. The teaching processes and learning experiences that must take place to achieve competency is left to the design of the curriculum developers and instructors.

TABLE 2
First Case Example

A Common Problem That Seemed to Defy the Right Approach to Solving It

---

A 52-year-old female, status posthysterectomy for endometrial cancer, presents with shortness of breath.
- High pretest probability of pulmonary embolism (PE): suggestive symptoms, major risk factors, and omission of appropriate perioperative venous thromboembolism (VTE) prophylaxis.
- Her presentation complicated by emesis, hypotension, hypoxia after presumed aspiration, and likely PE.
- Chest computed tomography (CT), PE protocol, reportedly negative for PE but positive for multilobar pneumonia.
- Small bowel obstruction, 51% bandemia, and acute renal failure.
- Subsequent emergency incarcerated hernia repair without VTE prophylaxis.
She is transferred to general medicine for hemodynamic monitoring and evaluation of hemoptysis and elevated troponin, presumably caused by a PE.
- Transthoracic echocardiogram notable for right ventricular (RV) dilation and pulmonary hypertension.
- Review of two chest CT scans, one PE protocol significant for an enlarged right ventricle and multilobar pneumonia but no PE.
- Absence of confirmatory evidence of suspected PE by subsequent extensive testing, including beta-natriuretic peptide (BNP) level, repeat PE protocol CT, repeat transthoracic echocardiogram, bilateral lower extremity ultrasound, persantine positron emission tomography (PET) scan, cardiac magnetic resonance imaging (MRI), and right heart catheterization.
- Discharge plan: home on warfarin.
- Repetitive testing did not alter management.
Retrospective review: Using the enlarged right atrium and ventricle as the radiographic clue to look more closely for PE, an experienced chest radiologist was able to diagnose the presence of acute PE on the first chest CT.

---

to prevent predictable complications of acute illness. Competencies in the Systems Organization and Improvement section indicate mastery of multiple competencies across categories. The Core Competencies describes how the hospitalist approach facilitates coordination among all participants within the hospital system (clinical and nonclinical) and effects system changes that improve patient care processes. At the same time, the statements indicate a range of involvement from participation to leadership. For example, "lead, coordination or participate in" acknowledges the unique needs of different practice settings and suggests a potential professional evolution. The Systems Organization and Improvement competencies of each clinical and procedure chapter strive to capture the essence of hospitalists whose goals are to improve patient outcomes for a specific population of patients. Hospitalists do not solely focus on the care of the patient with *x* disease, but rather develop systems to provide the best and most efficient care for *all* patients with *x* disease, successfully transitioning these patients to outpatient care and avoiding readmission.

The third section of chapters in the Core Competencies, Healthcare Systems, distinguishes a hospitalist from others working in the inpatient setting whether practicing at academic medical centers, community hospitals, teaching hospitals, managed-care settings, or for-profit settings. The Healthcare Systems section identifies the integral

components of the successful practice of hospital medicine and mastery of multiple competencies. This section highlights how hospitalists can facilitate coordination among all care providers within the hospital and with outpatient care providers. Hospitalists can effect system changes that improve complex care processes. It is likely that additional work experience and training beyond residency are required to attain global proficiency in the care of hospital medicine patients.

HOW TO USE THE CORE COMPETENCIES TO DEVELOP A CURRICULUM

The whole document, three sections and 51 chapters, develops expectations about the role of the hospitalist. Proficiency can be acquired through multiple means and should match the needs of the targeted learners in order to develop and maintain the necessary level of performance within the discipline of hospital medicine. Specific cases that hospitalists may encounter in their daily practice are used to illustrate how the Core Competencies can be applied to curriculum development.

The cases will employ the following six-step approach described in *Curriculum Development in Medical Education*[14]:

1. A problem and a need for improvement (the actual case and quality gap)
2. Needs assessment of targeted learners (hospitalists, clinicians-in-training)

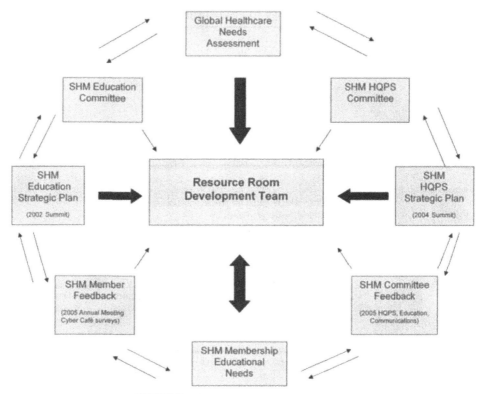

FIGURE 1. VTE resource room development process.

3. Goals and specific measurable objectives (with competencies bridging the gap between traditional roles and setting expectations about the hospitalist role)
4. Educational strategies (with competencies providing structure and guidance to educational efforts)
5. Implementation (applying competencies to a variety of training opportunities and curricula)
6. Evaluation and feedback (ongoing nationally, regionally, locally).

Like any quality-improvement educational initiative, subsequent steps in curriculum development for hospitalists should include, after evaluation and feedback, dissemination of core competencies and promotion of rigorous ongoing evaluation and adaptation as needs and expectations evolve.

The first case example, failure to prevent and diagnose pulmonary embolism (see Table 2), illustrates quality issues relating to prevention of predictable complications of illness, clinical problem solving in complex conditions of uncertainty, repetitive and nondiagnostic testing, and triage of a critically ill patient between services. The Core Competencies sets expectations about the ideal role of

the hospitalist that might lead to improved outcomes.

Using this case example, the Evidence-Based Medicine (EBM) chapter establishes explicit expectations for hospitalists in clinical problem solving, including 1) explaining how the tests help to verify a suspected diagnosis, 2) describing the human factor in test interpretation (e.g., technical limitations of the most recent multi-detector-row spiral CT), and 3) explaining how timing relative to the onset of symptoms affects test results. Rather than an overreliance on technology, leading to repeating the chest CT with PE protocol and subsequent excessive nondiagnostic testing, the hospitalist would use knowledge of pretest probability and test characteristics to determine the best diagnostic strategy. The hospitalist approach to patient care, articulated in the affective (attitudes) domains of each chapter, integrates the application of EBM principles to clinical problem solving with deliberation of cost effectiveness and efficiency.

Continuing with this case example, the Team Approach and Communication chapters establish explicit expectations for practicing hospitalists who

FIRST CASE EXAMPLE: APPLYING THE CORE COMPETENCIES TO CURRICULUM DEVELOPMENT

STEP 1
The current problem and the need for improvement

Quality Issues
- Prevention of predictable complications of illness: VTE still underutilized.
- Clinical problem-solving in complex systems, cost-effective, diagnostic testing.
- Triage of patients between services.

STEP 2
Needs assessment of hospitalists and other members of the inpatient team

The Current Approach: The focus of traditional medical education.
- How to manage a specific disease rather than how to manage complex patients with multiple co-morbidities.
- Didactic lectures on the pathophysiology of VTE .rather than prevention, QI.
- Individual feedback, morbidity and mortality conferences

STEP 3
Goals and specific measurable objectives

The Ideal Approach: Competencies as a framework for setting expectations about the role of the hospitalist
- Direct therapy against predictable complications of serious illness.
- Critically review prophylaxis.
- Devise strategies to bridge the gap between knowledge and practice.

STEP 4
Educational strategies

The first in a new online series: *The VTE Resource Room*, by SHM
- Key knowledge, approaches, methods, and tools can be applied to improve performance despite variances due to particular systems and advances in medicine.
- Enhance the ability of hospitalists as self-directed learners to improve inpatient outcomes.

STEP 5
Implementation

The VTE Resource Room
- A downloadable workbook and companion project outline for the improvement process.
- A slide set to disseminate valuable information about a safer system for VTE prevention.
- A moderated forum of VTE and QI experts to pose questions.

STEP 6
Evaluation and feedback

Ongoing Evaluation and Feedback
- Continuous with other steps (see Fig. 1).

STEP 7
Remaining questions—the need for additional research

Research Questions
- Identifying barriers to VTE prophylaxis in the hospital setting.
- Root cause analysis to determine prevention, process improvements, and training practices to encourage the safety of hospitalized patients.

TABLE 3
Second Case Example

The Hand-Off: Avoiding Pitfalls in the Hospitalist System

A 30-year-old female, status post–ruptured uterus and caesarian section for pregnancy, presents with hypotension.
- Shortness of breath post–exploratory laparoscopy during fluid resuscitation.
- Spiral CT performed to rule out pulmonary embolism, signed out as "negative" based on verbal report.
- Estimated pulmonary arterial systolic pressure of 70 mmHg by transthoracic echocardiogram.
- Extensive testing for underlying causes of pulmonary hypertension, hypercoagulable states.
- Outpatient right heart catheterization scheduled by cardiology.
- Sleep study advised to complete the workup of pulmonary hypertension.

After diuresis with a corresponding reduction in pulmonary capillary wedge pressure, her pulmonary hypertension resolves and her outpatient right heart catheterization is cancelled.
- Final reading of chest CT (not signed out to receiving attending) reportedly notable for moderate right-sided pleural effusion, small left-sided effusion, and an apparent filling defect of right subclavian vein
- Six days after the original spiral CT, unsuccessful thoracentesis attempted, with removal of 1 cc of fluid consistent with exudate.
- Video-assisted thoracoscopic surgery (VATS) procedure required to avoid chronic disability from trapped lung.

Retrospective review: Early drainage of a parapneumonic infection in the setting of sepsis might have avoided this complication.

SECOND CASE EXAMPLE: APPLYING THE CORE COMPETENCIES TO CURRICULUM DEVELOPMENT

STEP 1
The current problem and the need for improvement

Quality issues in the transfer of care.
- Failure to review radiographic study.
- Signing out pending test results.
- Failure to correlate imaging abnormalities with the patient's clinical presentation.

STEP 2
Seeds assessment of hospitalists and other embers of the inpatient team

The Current Approach: Inherent discontinuities of inpatient care.
- ACGME legislated work hours: resident shifts.
- Transfer of care to and from primary care physicians to hospitalists and between hospitalists.

STEP 3
Goals and specific measurable objectives

The Ideal Approach: Development of a standardized method of communication between hospitalists and between residents.
- A hand-off checklist would include pending tests, including final readings of radiographic studies.
- Systematic review of all films with a radiologist.

STEP 4
Educational strategies

Critical examination of local practice for variability in sign-outs.
- Development of curricula with an agreed-upon standard using the Core Competencies as a template—the Patient Hand-Offs chapter.
- Measure quality of hand-off and provide feedback.

STEP 5
Implementation

Dissemination of the expectations of the hand-off.
- Series of didactic talks for residents, physician assistants, and medical students by hospitalists based on specific cases.[19]
- Using the core competencies as a framework; didactic lectures on hospital medicine topics can be revised to better reflect the continuing educational needs of hospitalists and their roles and responsibilities.

STEP 6
Evaluation and feedback

A Framework for Educational Scholarship: the process of evaluation.
- Innovative educational pilots, designed for members of the multidisciplinary care team
- Clear goals, adequate preparation, appropriate methods, significant results, effective presentation, and reflective critique.
- New curricular designs and materials development in topics not traditionally taught during medical school and residency such as patient hand-offs[20,21]
- Not limited to publication; educational scholarship can be funded through risk management and hospital-funded seed grants.

STEP 7
Remaining questions—the need for additional research

Research Questions
- What are the key components of the sign-out process?
- How can an electronic medical record or other system be utilized to standardize and improve the process?

---

would take the extra steps to communicate with multiple members of the care team. Knowledgeable about the hospital, the hospitalist would review the chest CT with a radiologist skilled in chest interpretation and specifically query about the significance of an enlarged right atrium and right ventricle in the setting of a high pretest clinical probability of PE. Together the radiologist and hospitalist would consider a different imaging modality if the patient "flunked" the chest CT when the pretest probability was high. Rather than simply deferring to the medical specialist who is consulting, the hospitalist would be expected to improve the efficiency of care and reduce cost by only ordering tests that would change clinical management, perhaps with improved outcomes.

The Hospitalist as Teacher chapter provides a framework—core competencies for impromptu learning—based on the patient encounter. Members of the multidisciplinary care team can be exposed to explicit clinical decision making, an approach made possible by hospitalists on site, who can provide teaching moments in real time when decisions have to be made and educational feedback is needed. Teaching expectations for hospitalists include unambiguous clinical problem solving at the bedside and possibly directing the education of residents, physician assistants, and nurses on how to initiate a quality improvement (QI) project in a hospital setting.

The Quality Improvement and Venous Thromboembolism chapters clarify the role of the hospi-

TABLE 4
Third Case Example

'No Problem'

A proposal has been made that a new academic hospitalist service care for neurosurgical patients in order to meet the goals of the neurosurgical residency program to maximize the operating room exposure of surgeons in training.
- Patients would be admitted to the hospitalist service, with subsequent neurosurgical consultation.
- Another proposal has been made that the hospitalist service care for "uncovered patients" without residents in order to meet the goals of the medical residency program.
- Hospital leaders assume the hospitalist service would have no problem with this proposal.
- The hospitalists, who are not in-house at night, are asked to handle off-hours triage issues when there is disagreement between two services; their proposed role would be to support the medical residents who do not feel empowered to say "no" to the surgical team seeing patients in the emergency department.

The hospitalist service has the following concerns:
- Assuming responsibility for a nonteaching service undermines the vision of this new hospitalist service in an academic tertiary care facility.
- Assuming responsibility for a surgical specialty service increases medical legal risk and concerns about timely backup.
- Setting a bad precedent sends the wrong message.
- Hospitalists functioning as "superresidents" damages the reputation of the service.
- The proposal comes with a price, namely, accelerating physician burnout, declining job satisfaction, and inevitable turnover.
- The proposal would adversely affect future physician recruitment and promotion through the medical school clinician educator track.

Existing problems with the work environment of this new hospitalist service include:
- The service already does not have time to meet the responsibilities of inpatient care expected of hospitalists because of rapid growth and the need for further recruitment.
- Lack of advocacy by hospital administrators who may not understand the role of the hospitalist and entertain other solutions is an ongoing concern.
- Lack of support for other missions of teaching and quality improvement research, coupled with a changing job description and the daily unpredictability of the work, promotes the view that hospital medicine may not be sustainable as a career.

The challenge and opportunity: Expertise in strategic planning and operations management is needed in order to effectively respond to conflicting pressures and focus on goals that will sustain the ability to change, grow, and continuously improve.

---

talist, who should direct therapy against predictable complications of serious illness, critically review prophylaxis, provide hospital-specific data to clinicians, identify and lower barriers to prevention, devise strategies to bridge the gap between knowledge and practice, develop automated reminder systems, and participate in clinical research.

The SHM has used the Core Competencies to develop educational resources to better meet the needs of the healthcare system. Although patient safety initiatives are mandated by JCAHO for hospital accreditation and AHRQ has identified areas for safety improvement that lists venous thromboembolism (VTE) prevention as the number one priority, VTE prophylaxis is still underutilized in the United States. Although some mechanisms are in place to educate residents and hospitalists about how to manage a specific disease, traditional medical education does not focus on teaching students and residents how to manage complex patients with multiple comorbidities, to prevent predictable complications of illness, and to examine and improve care processes.[15,16] When it comes to leading quality improvement (QI), individual feedback and traditional curricula, which may include didactic lectures on the pathophysiology of VTE and mor-

bidity and mortality conferences, have not demonstrated improved outcomes.[17]

The SHM QI Web-based resource rooms offer support to any QI effort and raise collective awareness of a performance gap.[18] Each resource room will describe the evidence-based practices that should be put into effect and will leverage experience with the disease as well as with the improvement process. The underlying goal of the resource rooms is to enhance the ability of hospitalists to actually improve inpatient outcomes through self-directed learning (see Fig. 1).

Hospitalists, residency directors, and directors of hospitalist fellowships and continuing education can use *The Core Competencies in Hospital Medicine* to develop curricula for their local hospitalist service and request that invited speakers develop learning objectives and content based on core competencies rather than giving a prepared lecture on a specific clinical condition. This case of PE illustrates that risk assessment, prophylaxis, EBM clinical problem solving, and QI are core topics that should be emphasized in the training of hospitalists and physicians in training.

The second case example, the hand-off (see Table 3), illustrates quality issues related to transfer

STEP 1 The current problem and the need for improvement	Hospitalist Services cannot succeed by attempting to offer all things to all people. ● Distracting members from their work and from concentrating on their goals. ● Always saying "yes" to whoever asks for help as a Band-Aid, a short-term fix that impedes the effort and creativity required for durable long-term solutions to problems.
STEP 2 Needs assessment of hospitalists and other members of the inpatient team	*The Current Approach:* Problems with the work environment ● Hospital medicine, a new specialty, does not yet have a similar supportive infrastructure analogous to other well-established specialties with most hospitalist programs within divisions of general medicine. ● Multiple stakeholders—administrators, primary care providers, residency and clerkship directors, specialty services. ● Leadership and administrative skills are not consistently acquired proficiencies during residency training.
STEP 3 Goals and specific measurable objectives	*The Ideal Approach:* Hospitalists can proactively improve their work life by developing skills and knowledge in hospital systems. ● Develop personal, team, and program goals. ● Identify and resolve conflicts using specific negotiation techniques ● Enhance program development and growth. ● Identify senior physician leaders as mentors and advocates.
STEP 4 Educational strategies	Annual retreats to generate enthusiasm, establish a strategic plan, continue a trajectory of success. ● Invite an outside expert in QI or professional development to facilitate discussion. ● Recruit hospitalists and colleagues with expertise in healthcare systems to mentor and educate other members of the hospitalist service how to lead QI and other initiatives.
STEP 5 Implementation	Use the core competencies to advocate for resources to support professional goals. ● Funding for leadership courses and further training in business. ● Directors of CME sponsored by SHM have begun the process of using the core competencies as the framework for the development of hospital medicine curricula in leadership and QI.
STEP 6 Evaluation and feedback	Consider using the Core Competencies to develop an internal report card on performance. ● A self-assessment tool based on the core values and goals of the hospitalist program. ● A means to help identify areas for improvement, modifiable risk factors for turnover, and opportunities to provide incentives to measure interventions, reward success, and ultimately deliver on the mandate to improve inpatient care.
STEP 7 Remaining questions—the need for additional research	Challenges facing hospitalists practicing in multiple settings. ● How to make processes of care efficient by examining specific tasks that hospitalists do and determining what tools, technologies, organizational structure, and supporting staff need to be available to make the performance of these tasks efficient. ● How to make hospital medicine a sustainable and satisfying career.

of care from one physician to another. In this example, if the patient with moderate pleural effusion had been signed out, an earlier thoracentesis to drain a presumptive parapneumonic infection might have relieved this patient's shortness of breath and saved her from undergoing a subsequent VATS procedure. This case also demonstrates the importance of correlating imaging abnormalities with a patient's clinical presentation rather than using the traditional approach of just "ruling out" potential diagnoses to determine the cause of a problem. This case highlights elements of the process and system of care that can be modified to

improve patient outcomes. Being proficient in transferring care of patients can save the hospitalist from error and prevent adverse events.

The Team Approach chapter establishes the need to acquire proficiencies not ordinarily obtained during residency in order to lead a multidisciplinary care team. This role requires a level of functioning beyond that of simply being the attending of record. The hospitalist must be able to synthesize information rather than simply defer to the consultant. Competencies specified in the Diagnostic Decision-Making chapter can be used to identify the educational needs of hospitalists, who are expected to minimize diagnostic errors by knowing when to ask for help and where to get it, recognizing common diseases with uncommon presentations, and generating a broad differential diagnosis where there is uncertainty. The Patient Handoff chapter defines the proficiencies hospitalists need to facilitate the safe transfer of patients to other physicians on their service.

The third case example, which expands the responsibilities of hospitalist to include meeting important needs in the hospital (see Table 4), illustrates that hospitalist services cannot succeed by offering all things to all people, a distraction that that keeps the members of these services from concentrating on their goals. Always saying "yes" to whoever asks for help is a band-aid, a short-term fix that impedes the effort and creativity required for durable long-term solutions to problems.

The Core Competencies sets expectations about the roles of hospitalists, who serve as well-informed clinicians and clinical opinion leaders; effective educators, mentors, and role models; empathetic and timely communicators; efficient caregivers; and creative problem solvers arriving at durable, longer-term solutions. The competencies demonstrate the knowledge, skills, and attitudes required to be effective agents of change. Changing business as usual almost always requires significant improvements in the underlying system, however uncomfortable. The Leadership chapter articulates competencies that hospitalists need in order to define their roles within the hospital, promote group cohesiveness, expand their practices intelligently, and anticipate and respond to change. This chapter details the proficiencies that hospitalists need in order to develop personal, team, and program goals and to identify and resolve conflicts using specific negotiation techniques. The Business Practices chapter articulates the fundamental skills needed to enhance program development and growth. Hospitalists can use the Core Competencies to identify educational needs and develop curricula to enhance their leadership and business skill sets.

Medical educators should examine the outcomes of current training practices and assess what modifications of objectives, content, and instructional strategies should be made to better prepare the current and next generations of physicians to practice hospital medicine and to improve the hospital setting. Given the scope of the field of hospital medicine, the Core Competencies should guide: 1) what to teach and how much to teach; 2) how to teach and assess trainees, and how to assess and compare faculty development programs; 3) how to design systems for improving quality of care and assuring patient safety; and 4) how to establish priorities for hospital medicine research.

TRANSLATING A SET OF COMPETENCIES INTO CURRICULA: POTENTIAL BENEFITS

The Core Competencies in Hospital Medicine transcends hospital type, size, and setting and standardizes what the expectations for and proficiencies of a practicing hospitalist should be. By defining the role of the hospitalist, the Core Competencies serves as a resource for refining inpatient skills and assists in program development at the local, regional, and national levels. In addition, by using the Core Competencies as the standard and framework for the development of preparatory curricula, hospital administrators and other employers can rely on hospitalists having had a common preparation.

The medical profession is constantly evolving. Internal medicine curricula address the challenges hospital medicine physicians faced yesterday but could improve the training and preparation of physicians to serve in their new and emerging roles as leaders of multidisciplinary healthcare teams working to improve patient outcomes and the system of inpatient care. Hospital medicine no longer represents a group of physicians merely supporting other specialists and primary care physicians; it is itself a specialty, composed of physicians leading, directing, and improving inpatient care. The competencies presented in *The Core Competencies in Hospital Medicine: A Framework for Curriculum Development*, by the Society of Hospital Medicine, should spark debate about the adequacy and appropriateness of current training and certification expectations and serve as a foundation for the development of curricula to improve hospital medicine education.

Address for correspondence and reprint requests: Sylvia C. W. McKean, MD, FACP, Medical Director, Brigham and Women's Faulkner Hospitalist Service, Harvard Medical School, Boston, MA; Fax: (617) 264-5137; E-mail: smckean@partners.org

Received 26 August 2005; revision received 7 November 2005; accepted 14 November 2005.

REFERENCES

1. Wachter RM, Goldman L. The emerging role of "hospitalists" in the American health care system. *N Engl J Med.* 1996;335:514–517.
2. Wachter RM, Goldman L. The hospitalist movement 5 years later. *JAMA.* 2002;287:487–494.

3. Kelley MA. The hospitalist: a new medical specialty? *Ann Intern Med.* 1999;130:373–375.
4. Pistoria MJ, Amin AN, Dressler DD, McKean SCW, Budnitz TL, eds. *The Core Competencies in Hospital Medicine: A Framework for Curriculum Development. J Hosp Med.* 2006;1 (supplement 1).
5. Dressler DD, Pistoria MJ, Budnitz TL, McKean SCW, Amin AN. Core competencies in hospital medicine: development and methodology. *J Hosp Med.* 2006;1:48–56.
6. Koh LT, Corrigan JM, Donaldson MS, eds. To err is human. Washington, DC: National Academy Press, 2000.
7. Shojania KG, Duncan BW, McDonald KM, Wachter RM, Markowitz AJ. Making healthcare safer: a critical analysis of patient safety practices. AHRQ publication 01-E058, 2001.
8. Joint Commission on the Accreditation of Health Care Organizations. Available at URL: http://www.jcaho.org [accessed November 2005].
9. Accreditation Council for Graduate Medical Education. Available at URL: http://www.acgme.org [accessed November 2005].
10. Ende J, Davidoff F. What is a curriculum? *Ann Intern Med.* 1992;116:1055–1056.
11. Ende J, Atkins E. Conceptualizing curriculum for graduate medical education. *Acad Med.* 1992;67:528–534.
12. American Association for Health Education, National Commission for Health Education Credentialing, Inc., Society for Public Health Education. A competency-based framework for graduate-level health educators. Allentown, PA: NCHEC, 1999.
13. Gronlund NE. How to write and use instructional objectives. 6th ed. Upper Saddle River, NJ: Prentice Hall, 2000.
14. Kern DE, Thomas PA, Howard DM, et al. Curriculum development for medical education: a six-step approach. Baltimore: Johns Hopkins University Press, 1998.
15. Ratnapalan S, Hilliard RI. Needs assessment in postgraduate medical education: a review. *Med Educ Online* [serial online]. 2002;7. Available at URL: http://www.med-ed-online.org/pdf/f0000040.pdf [accessed December 7, 2005].
16. Green M. Identifying, appraising, and implementing medical education curricula: a guide for medical educators. *Ann Intern Med.* 2001;135:889–896.
17. Kucher N, Koo S, Quiroz R, et al. A quality improvement initiative at Brigham and Women's Hospital. *N Engl J Med.* 2005;352:969.
18. The Society of Hospital Medicine. Available from URL: http://www.hospitalmedicine.org [accessed November 2005].
19. Barnes LB, Christensen CR, Hersen AJ. Teaching and the case method. 3rd ed. Cambridge, MA: Harvard Business School, 1994.
20. Boyer EL. Scholarship reconsidered: priorities of the professoriate. Princeton, NJ: Carnegie Foundation for the Advance of Teaching, 1990.
21. Hafler JP, Lovejoy FH Jr. Scholarly activities of faculty promoted in a teacher–clinician ladder. *Acad Med.* 2000;75:649–52.